Measuring Health Care

Yosef D. Dlugacz

Measuring Health Care

Using Data for Operational, Financial, and Clinical Improvement

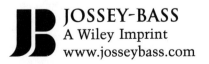

JOSSEY-BASS
A Wiley Imprint
www.josseybass.com

Published by Jossey-Bass
A Wiley Imprint
989 Market Street, San Francisco, CA 94103-1741   www.josseybass.com

Jossey-Bass books and products are available through most bookstores. To contact Jossey-Bass directly call our Customer Care Department within the U.S. at 800-956-7739, outside the U.S. at 317-572-3986, or fax 317-572-4002.

Jossey-Bass also publishes its books in a variety of electronic formats. Some content that appears in print may not be available in electronic books.

Library of Congress Cataloging-in-Publication Data
Dlugacz, Yosef D., 1947–
  Measuring health care : using data for operational, financial, and clinical improvement / Yosef D. Dlugacz.
    p. ; cm.
  Includes bibliographical references and index.
  ISBN-13: 978-0-7879-8383-3 (pbk.)
  ISBN-10: 0-7879-8383-7 (pbk.)
    1. Medical care. 2. Medical care—Utilization. 3. Medicine
—Research—Data processing. 4. Medical care, Cost of. 5. Medi-
cal care—Quality control. I. Title.
    [DNLM: 1. Data Collection—methods—United States. 2. Quality
Assurance, Health Care—methods—United States. 3. Outcome
Assessment (Health Care)—United States. W 84 AA1 D626m
2006]
  RA395.A3D558 2006
  362.1068—dc22
                                                   2006014167

Printed in the United States of America
FIRST EDITION
PB Printing   10 9 8 7 6 5 4 3 2 1

~~~ Contents

To my beloved family—Doris, who has stood by my side every step of the way, and Adam, Stacey, Stefanie, and Hillel, who provide me with endless support and joy.

—ᴡᴡ— Figures and Tables

Figures

—ᴧᴧ— Preface

I am writing this book to fill what I perceive as a critical gap in information. For health care to survive in this country, by which I mean for health care institutions to provide excellent patient care and also remain profitable, individuals who are involved with health care policy formulation and health care administration need to understand the value of data and use data as the basis for delivering quality care and achieving financial success.

My previous book, *The Quality Handbook for Health Care Organizations,* was a practical primer on how to integrate quality management methods into various aspects of the delivery of care. As I travel across the country introducing these quality concepts to health care professionals, I am struck with how little they know about using indicators and measurements—even though they are required to collect and analyze information from these quality tools. With this book my hope is to convince health care leaders that measures must be the basis of informed decisions and that without appropriate measures there can be no real oversight of hospital processes and operations. Most important, without measures there can be no real improvements in health care services.

Measuring Health Care is the product of my twenty years of working with quality management. I began, as most quality managers then did, as the person responsible for interpreting governmental regulatory standards for busy clinicians, who generally found compliance with the standards an annoyance. Over the years, as health care has become ever more complex, as quality management has evolved, and as the organization where I work (the North Shore–Long Island Jewish Health System) has expanded to include not only more hospitals but also nursing homes, rehabilitation facilities, a children's hospital, and a behavioral health facility, my understanding of what managing quality means has evolved as well.

As a sociologist, I was trained to ask questions, sometimes hard questions, and to use data to discover the answers. I accompanied caregivers on the units, I sat in the emergency departments, and I spoke to the cleaning staff. My goal was to understand how the hospital functioned and also the relationship between providing excellent clinical care and an efficient operation.

I was extremely fortunate, as were our patients, that the individuals who served on the board of trustees wanted to understand that relationship as well, and they looked to me to explain it to them. When I presented quality measures to them, they were smart enough to ask what those numbers meant and why those numbers were interesting, and they were caring enough to wonder how they could use this information to make the hospital better. They were right on the money: information in a vacuum is meaningless. Information without context, without a methodology for improvement, without a vision for the organization, is just isolated bits of data.

As I struggled to answer their questions about the provision of care and its relationship to operational success, I realized that I needed more information. I needed to carefully define variables of quality to understand what I was measuring and monitoring, and I needed to standardize those definitions across the various institutions of the health system if I were going to aggregate and track and trend the data being collected and if I were to be able to answer the trustees' questions.

The quality management department was expanded; along with more quality managers, analysts and statisticians were hired. Before long, working in quality involved far more than translating regulatory requirements and monitoring compliance for accreditation. Quality had become what it is designed to be—an objective definition of the delivery of service and a methodology that could be integrated into every aspect of the health care institution so that each aspect could be evaluated, understood, and improved.

This book, *Measuring Health Care,* is the result of my experience over the past twenty years. For me, it has been an incredibly rewarding personal journey. I fervently believe in the quality management philosophy, and I have a tremendous respect for its methodology, which, when applied, has produced enormous improvements in patient safety and organizational success. Because I am such a champion of quality, I am asked to teach its principles to professional and managerial staffs and to students of business and health in graduate colleges across the country. I teach from my experience, with examples from my work. My goal is to incorporate the objectivity and evaluative criteria of quality tools, techniques, and philosophy into the fabric of care. In this book I hope to teach the reader what I teach my students and to do it in the same way—with examples and with information and with commitment to the process.

It all begins with measures.

ACKNOWLEDGMENTS

This book could not have been written without the help and experience of many others. I am especially grateful to the members of the North Shore–Long Island Jewish Health System board of trustees, who believed in quality and generously contributed their wisdom and their time to ensuring that the health system continuously strives toward excellence.

I also want to express my particular gratitude to long-time trustee Abe Krasnoff, who for many years has made it clear that he believes not only in quality and in measurements but also in me. His commitment and generosity in funding the Julienne and Abraham Krasnoff Center for Advanced Studies in Quality, which I direct, underlines his confidence in the quality process. Thank you, Abe.

I want to thank the chairs of the Joint Conference Professional Affairs Committees, who worked tirelessly and often thanklessly to pursue our quality goals: Howard Stave, chair, Acute Care and Behavioral Health; Stuart Levine, chair, Ambulatory Care; Edwin Stein, chair, Long Term Care, Rehabilitation, Home Care, and Hospice; and Frank Scarangello, chair, Safety and Environment of Care. To them, to the members of the committees, and to Mark Claster, chair, of the Committee on Quality, I owe a great deal.

Michael J. Dowling, president and CEO of the North Shore–Long Island Jewish Health System, promotes an organization that values quality and measurements. His leadership and support have encouraged me to develop the tools needed to express complex phenomena so that quality information can be used for daily operations. For that and for the opportunity to teach others about quality management I am grateful.

A special thank-you goes to Dr. Abdallah S. Mishrick, an extraordinary and much missed medical and surgical leader whose passion, integrity, and energy continue to inspire me personally and professionally.

The existence of this book owes a great deal to the outstanding professionals who make up the Quality Management Department: Andrea Restifo, my right hand, whose intelligence and love of quality have enabled me to do my best work; Karen Nelson, who shares my passion for the importance of data; and Marcella DeGeronimo and her analysts Karen Miller and Roshan Hussain, who produce magnificent reports.

And to the rest of the superb staff I am fortunate to work with, much thanks. Thanks to the graphic designers, Rico Rosales and Hillel Dlugacz, who work magic with computer design and art. Thanks also to Debi Baker, whose administrative skill was invaluable in producing this book, and to Joyce Guerriere, whose loyalty and support keep me going every day.

The folks at Jossey-Bass, Andy Pasternack and his team, have made this process a pleasure. Thanks for your support of this work from the beginning.

Finally, I must thank Alice Greenwood, my colleague and my friend, who translates my thoughts into words.

May 2006   Yosef D. Dlugacz
                                                     Great Neck, New York

⟶ The Author

YOSEF D. DLUGACZ, senior vice president of quality management for the North Shore–Long Island Jewish Health System, is responsible for oversight of that organization's extensive quality management program, which spans a broad and diverse spectrum of services and facilities. As dean of the system's Center for Learning and Innovation, he has educated many professionals in quality management and measurements.

Dlugacz is also the professional faculty coordinator for Hofstra University's M.B.A. program and has lectured at Albert Einstein Hospital in Brazil and at Georgetown University. He is adjunct research professor at New York University and visiting professor at Beijing University's M.B.A. program. He serves on the board of directors of the American Heart Association and is a consultant for the Council on Accreditation of the College of American Pathologists. He is on the faculty of the Healthcare Association of New York State (HANYS) Data Academy and is a member of the HANYS steering committee and the American Medical Association clinical measures workgroup.

In 2004, Dlugacz was named director of the Julienne and Abraham Krasnoff Center for Advanced Studies in Quality. Many of the best practices developed under his supervision have been published by the Joint Commission on Accreditation of Healthcare Organizations as setting standards for the entire health care industry. He has published widely in health care and quality management journals on a variety of clinical care and quality topics. His previous book, *The Quality Handbook for Health Care Organizations: A Manager's Guide to Tools and Programs* (Jossey-Bass, 2004), is being used as a text for both clinical and financial programs in quality management and as a practical training tool for health care professionals.

Dlugacz holds a doctorate in sociology from the City University of New York.

─ɷ─ Introduction

Health care in the United States is in crisis. No other country spends as much money as ineffectively and as inefficiently as we do. Insurance premiums are rising while coverage is shrinking. It's estimated that over 42 million Americans are uninsured and have little access to adequate health services. Clearly, something is seriously wrong. Health care services are not meeting the needs of the people. The solutions that have been put forth by the government and policy-makers have not addressed the underlying problems in what is clearly a broken system.

One of the most fundamental questions to be addressed to improve the situation is deceptively simple: How do we know when health care services are "good"? The answer, also simple, is to measure those services. Another basic question is this: Is health care fair in terms of access and cost? The answer, again, is measures. When measures are used to analyze how health care institutions perform in quality and in finance, the organization has a basis for understanding its delivery of care and for improving that care.

Individuals who are interested in understanding the complex issues related to health care policy, health care administration, health services management, and quality management require education about new trends in monitoring health care and about ways to interpret the financial viability of health care services. Among these new trends is the idea of defining health care as a *product,* a commodity available for the public to purchase. For the first time in history, these purchasing decisions are being based on objective standards of evaluation that are communicated in various ways and through various forums. Quality indicators are being introduced to the public as evaluative barometers of health care delivery and to health care organizations as standards for accreditation and financial reimbursement.

The purpose of *Measuring Health Care: Using Data for Operational, Financial, and Clinical Improvement* is to educate those who work in health care services or management, health care administration, public health policy, and business administration about how to develop, define, understand, use, evaluate, and react to the various kinds of measures. Because measures underlie all quality management, the basic tenets of quality management will be explained. This book will inform leaders of health care organizations and students of health care services about using measures to influence and monitor patient safety, quality of care, and organizational success and will help them understand how to collect and interpret statistical information and respond to governmental oversight. Quality measures should be used to guide strategic planning, to improve financial performance, to formulate policies, and to move health care into the future.

Just as administrators know how to react to deficits noted in financial reports, they should know how to respond appropriately when a quality indicator is used to report a problem. They need to know what it means, how this piece of information interacts with other indicators, what it reveals about the care delivered in the health care institution, and how the problem can be addressed and improved. This book will help administrators learn to use measures to ask the right questions of the professional staff and understand how to interpret the answers. Measures can be used to reduce the separation and the conflict among physicians, administrators, governance, regulatory agencies, patients, and payers.

Measuring Health Care: Using Data for Operational, Financial, and Clinical Improvement is designed to inform health care professionals how to use databases and quality management tools and techniques to best purpose; to analyze care, services, safety, and appropriateness; and to make meaningful financial decisions for organizational success. Armed with an understanding of quality indicators, administrators will be able to break down the wall between clinical practice and financial viability. Through overseeing and understanding databases that include quality management indicators, utilization management indicators, safety indicators, and environmental indicators, health care leaders will be able to improve communication among various administrative and clinical departments to the benefit of both the institution and the patients it serves.

As senior vice president of a large health care system, I bring twenty years of experience in quantitative analysis for performance improvement in health care to this discussion. In this personal, practical, and hands-on approach to improving care, I use hypothetical case studies, compiled from actual events, to illustrate how measures can and should be used to monitor organizational effectiveness. I explain the process of acquiring valid data, the methods to use to interpret data in order for the delivery of care to be accurately analyzed, and the role of data in designing and improving processes of care and in developing financial success.

This book is organized by topics, with each chapter addressing measurements related to clinical, organizational, and financial goals. Case examples are offered to illustrate how the theory translates into practice. At the end of each chapter I offer "things to think about." These exercises are designed to focus on the central ideas presented in the chapter and to be adaptable for people in differing educational and professional areas.

Chapter One presents an overview of the major themes that will be developed throughout the rest of the book and exposes the reader to general information about the ways in which measures have an impact on the health care organization and its medical staff, patients, leadership, finance, and evaluation of care.

Chapter Two reviews the fundamentals of data, stressing the importance of combining quality and financial data into organizational and clinical reports. Basic concepts related to quality management are explained, in particular how to use data to understand the delivery of care and to gauge improvements. Case examples reveal how data analysis can inform patient care. Different formats for communicating quality data are discussed, their use depending on leadership goals and on levels of accountability for improvements.

In Chapter Three principles of evidence-based medicine are presented, along with the role of measures in defining the standard of care. I discuss considering health care as a marketable consumer product and ways in which measures can be used to understand consumer needs and improve market share. The financial implications of measures for good clinical care and the importance to administrative leadership are also discussed.

Chapter Four outlines quality management methodology and how to use measures for performance improvement. The numerators and denominators of measures can be developed to monitor specific areas of interest, depending on leadership priorities and goals. Once measures are defined and tracked over time, administrative leadership can use the information as a basis for purchasing and other financial decisions. The Plan Do Check Act (PDCA) methodology for performance improvement is also explained, with a case example showing the method in practice.

In Chapter Five I discuss how measures can be used for preventive oversight for patient safety, which in turn results in improved organizational efficiency. Measures of clinical and organizational efficiency should also be used when communicating with the governing body, the board of trustees, to explain the delivery of care. One of the challenges for organizational leadership is to enlist the physicians to accept measures as definers of performance and quality and as a tool to increase their accountability, both to their patients and the organization. Methods of analyzing errors and adverse events are presented in this chapter, using data to assess care and make changes in the way physicians practice.

Chapter Six describes the external drivers of quality, those governmental and private agencies that dictate standards of care by determining the measures that hospitals have to meet in order to be accredited and receive financial incentives. Public pressure, consumer groups, and the media also have an impact on health care policy and on the way health care service is delivered. The role of quality management departments in mediating between the organization and these external groups is discussed here. The case example in this chapter illustrates how the public reporting of data can drive changed practices.

Chapter Seven offers examples of how to interpret report cards and how the relationship between quality and finance affects operations. I explain here the different sources and uses of administrative and primary data and how best to use these data to improve care and efficient operations. High-level reports of quality indicators, as a kind of executive summary, are discussed as a method of communicating complex information about quality measures and of tracking and trending information to identify best practices and to target opportunities for improvement.

In Chapter Eight I discuss the value of using clinical pathways and clinical guidelines to incorporate evidence-based standards into the delivery of care and to promote communication among the caregiving staff. Variance data, collected from the guidelines, help to identify gaps in the delivery of care for concurrent resolution. Retrospective and aggregated analysis of the guideline data reveals areas that require improvement. An outline of how to develop and promote clinical guidelines is offered in this chapter, and a case example again shows how theory can be put into practice.

Chapter Nine presents several performance improvement initiatives that incorporate the information from the previous chapters, illustrating how to use data for assessment and improvement and how to use the PDCA to continuously monitor success.

The Conclusion suggests next steps in the evolution of quality standards and medical care, in particular how to achieve physician acceptance and generate culture change.

Measuring Health Care

CHAPTER ONE

Overview

What Measures Measure

I magine that hospital rankings have just been released in the local newspapers and made available on the Web. Members of the health care organization's board of trustees begin calling its senior leadership and asking questions—hard questions, such as why wasn't the hospital's cardiac mortality rate the lowest in the state? They want to know what the problems are and what is being done to improve the situation. Chief executive officers (CEOs), senior leadership, and administrators often try to ignore the data and to assure the community that negative reports do not reflect what is actually happening in their hospital. They stress that their excellent, well-trained physicians and nurses are doing a great job. But this response is not always convincing in the face of the numbers.

Health care administrators, managers, policymakers, and executives are expected to have the information to respond intelligently to negative data. That's part of their job. In order to respond, they need to be able to use broad enough brush strokes to create a high level of understanding, yet they must also offer enough specific detail to encompass the complexity of the questions—and the answers.

If, for example, the news media report a high infection rate in a hospital, what does that mean? In other words, what exactly is the measure *infection rate* measuring? Interpreting such measures for the general public can be a challenge for health care leaders because the data that describe complex medical phenomena may not be congruent with the assumption that there is a straightforward relationship between cause (treatment) and effect (outcome). To understand this infection rate measure, leadership should have information about whether the problem is limited to one hospital unit or is running rampant across many units, or whether the infection is connected to a single procedure, physician, staff member, operating room, or technological process. Perhaps the infection occurs only in patients who have been transferred from a specific nursing home or who live in a particular neighborhood. Data can reveal whether the infection rate has increased over time (and if so, by how much) and can identify the group of patients or staff involved. Data can expose how severe the infection is, where the cases are located (which department or unit in the hospital), how long the length of stay (LOS) is for those patients with the infection, and what costs are associated with their care.

The data to address these and many other questions are available through quality management and various other databases, and health care leaders need to acquire the familiarity and skill to interpret the data and must also be able to communicate about the issues with the clinical staff, the media, and the community.

The successful health care professional is committed to running an efficient organization, and that entails understanding data from quality indicators and measurements and how these data can be used to link clinical results and policy formation. Because most administrators are concerned with how to do damage control when the public reads about poor outcomes in the local newspapers, it is essential that they become familiar with the dynamics of care and position themselves to introduce changes that will improve the reports—and the care.

Recently I attended a meeting of the medical board of a small community hospital and spoke to two staff cardiologists who were understandably upset that they both had fared poorly on the mortality ranking published in their local newspaper. They said they were reluctant to go to the supermarket because people were asking them questions they couldn't answer. These physicians didn't know what was wrong with the care they delivered and in fact were convinced that their care was excellent and that the rankings were faulty.

The CEO of the hospital, also being questioned, didn't know where to look for explanations of the high mortality. In such circumstances it is easy to make excuses: the coding was inaccurate; the patients were sicker than average, with complications; the physicians do great work but are too busy to document the charts and therefore the measure is a reflection merely of inaccurate paperwork and not the inadequate delivery of care. Excuses, which may calm some people in the supermarket, don't take the measure seriously, or worse, they prevent leadership and physicians from analyzing their processes, the delivery of services, or the gaps in their care. This denial and blame mentality does not lead to self-criticism or self-improvement. Outcomes analysis, such as an examination of the reasons for a high mortality rate, requires data that can explain a clinical phenomenon, such as death. Data can help to determine whether the intervention (or lack of it) contributed to the mortality or whether the existing clinical and organizational environment is appropriate for preventing poor outcomes.

Familiarity and comfort with quality measures encourage leaders, administrators, and policymakers to understand important variables in clinical areas as well as in organizational processes. Measures can focus attention on potential problem areas; measures can specify small issues before they result in major incidents; measures can monitor improvements. Most important, measures provide a method of communication among medical staff and hospital administrators.

MEASURES AND THE MEDICAL STAFF

Paradoxically, the very physicians on whom a measure depends do not always feel obligated to meet the expectations of that measure. For example, the federal government, through the Centers for Medicare and Medicaid Services (CMS), has developed a measure that is based on evidence from research, clinical trials, and medical expertise showing that patients suffering heart attacks (technically referred to as acute myocardial infarctions, or AMIs) have a more positive outcome when they receive an aspirin (ASA) within four hours of coming to the emergency department (ED). The CMS collects the data about the rate of aspirin administration to AMI patients in order to monitor, and one hopes improve, patient outcomes. However, it is the physician who controls whether or not a patient is administered an aspirin, and it is the physician's responsibility to document the medical record so that the CMS indicator can be aggregated for the hospital. Without physician acceptance the intent of this measure cannot be met.

The Centers for Medicare and Medicaid Services (CMS) is the governmental agency responsible for administering the Medicare program, and it also works with the states to administer Medicaid. In addition to providing health insurance, the CMS is involved in quality standards. State surveyors visit a number of health care organizations annually to determine compliance with CMS quality standards and to investigate complaints. The CMS contracts with medical organizations to ensure that the medical care paid for with Medicare funds is reasonable and necessary, meets professionally recognized standards, and is provided economically. The CMS is working to improve the quality of health care by measuring and improving outcomes of care, educating health care providers about quality improvement opportunities, and educating the public to make good health care choices.

Typically, administrators have relied on physicians to explain medical phenomena, and physicians have done so by discussing the characteristics of their patients' illnesses. However, more and more research points to the realization that explanations for medical phenomena can be found in aggregated data about global process issues and not solely in the analysis of individual patient problems. Measurements that reflect aggregated processes of care objectively, as well as outcomes of that care, help physicians move past their own patients to understand how to improve outcomes and performance for all patients.

In other words, measures can be used by administrators and physicians to generalize across the patient population and to develop policies and make decisions based on aggregated data. Measures can provide a common language for physicians and administrators by interpreting objective variables. Through a shared language—that is, the measures—a hospital can be transformed from a collection of groups with specific and differing agendas to an integrated working team with similar goals.

MEASURES AND PATIENTS

Patients today are reacting to the media attention to medical errors and the dangers involved in hospitalization. Having been informed by such an august body as the Institute of Medicine (IOM), an independent organization of medical experts who study the health care industry, that almost 100,000 deaths occur unnecessarily every year in the United States due to medical mistakes, the public is scared, where once it was trusting. Reinforcing this fear, the Institute for Healthcare Improvement (IHI) has launched a campaign to save 100,000 lives by enlisting hospitals to commit to implementing changes in care that would avoid preventable deaths. Although this campaign is laudable, it underlines the lack of patient safety in hospitals and the fact that senior administrators seem unable to fix existing problems that affect patient safety.

People have begun to approach health care services in a new way—informed, suspicious, and eager to take responsibility for their own care. Patients ask questions of their physicians and of health care leaders as they have never done before. Today's baby boomers are not about to settle for a patronizing pat on the head, and a leave-it-to-the-expert attitude that perhaps worked well in the world of their parents. Patients are eager to be well informed and to research solutions to their health care problems. They look further than their personal physicians for information. They find answers by examining the data available: how many procedures has a specific specialist performed; what was the mortality rate on those procedures, for the hospital and for the physician; how many disciplinary actions are recorded for the physician and how many malpractice claims? In addition, hospital and individual physician profiles are now available for public scrutiny. Public pressure is mounting, as can be seen by the increase in drug advertisements on television and in magazines, and by the technological innovations that patients demand as solutions to medical issues. These types of social forces shape organizational change.

The following selected Web sites provide information about health care services:

webapps.ama-assn.org/ doctorfinder	Provides background information and achievements and certifications of physicians

bestdoctors.com	Offers peer review of physicians who have met standards of care
compareyourcare.org	Rates quality of care with national guidelines
healthfinder.gov	Provides ratings of hospitals and nursing homes
healthgrades.com	Ranks physicians, hospitals, and nursing homes
jcaho.org	Presents comparison information for health care organizations
leapfroggroup.org	Reports on and compares hospital quality outcomes
ncqa.org	Ranks health plans, including information about their performance
qualitymeasures.ahrq.gov	Compares quality measures across institutions
ratemds.com	Provides patients' ratings of doctors

Responding to the needs and interests of the modern patient, the state and federal governments are providing the public with research-based information about appropriate disease management (evidence-based medicine) and making available algorithms of care—what should be done, when, why, and to whom. Patients are encouraged to partner in their health care decisions, to get second opinions, and to learn the details of appropriate expectations through informed consent forms that describe the risks and benefits of procedures. It is insufficient to provide patients with excellent, hotel-like services (as many institutions are now doing to try to bolster their patient satisfaction rates); the hospital must also be able to report good patient outcomes.

MEASURES AND HEALTH CARE LEADERS

In order to meet the new challenges head-on, today's health care professionals need to equip themselves to evaluate the *product* delivered in their organization. Through using measures an organization can prove that its product is *good,* reassuring the public about safety and thus maximizing revenue. Achieving this goal requires an understanding of how to measure, what to measure, how to interpret measures, and how to monitor care through measures on an ongoing basis. Most important, information from the analysis of measures should be applied to improve the delivery of care and increase patient safety.

For example, how would you, as a senior administrator, respond if the chief finance officer reports that the intensive care units (ICUs) are costing the hospital a fortune and should be reevaluated? What criteria should be used to make improvements and change practices? The physicians will tell you their patients need to be in an ICU because they require specialized care. Are they right? How would a nonclinician evaluate what the physicians say? Have standards been established for admission to the unit? Are there other units in the hospital that might be as appropriate for caregiving? Most important, are there any data to support the physicians' stance, or are any data available to indicate that expensive ICU care may not improve the health and well-being of their patients?

Of course health care managers and administrators are in no position to argue medical care with physicians. But they can put themselves in a position to understand utilization issues, to document the patient population, to develop policies about end-of-life care, to track the relationship between processes and outcomes, and to evaluate how money is being spent. If an administrator has data that show that the ICU is not necessary for patients to receive appropriate care, that the outcomes are the same in less resource-intensive units, that, for example, it is unnecessary for patients to be in an ICU while awaiting a stress test that could be administered in a physician's office, physicians and the governing body will take notice. Availability of data permits the administrator to see beyond the individual physician's patients and to evaluate the bigger organizational picture.

Professionals involved in health care administration, services, and policy formulation can ill afford to be uninformed; it puts them at too much of a disadvantage. Policy and financial decisions must be based on information, such as data describing the patient population or data defining appropriate levels of care based on acuity of illness or condition. Because medical care influences the budget, administrators and health care managers have to provide themselves with the tools and the education to understand that care. The separation of powers between the clinical and the administrative staff, typical of the late-twentieth century, is not useful today because a silo approach to information and communication cannot explain how care is delivered or improved, nor can outcomes be predicted.

Health care, like other industries, uses specific techniques to better the competitive edge, to increase production, so to speak, and maintain financial viability. Administrators need to use innovative methods for balancing the number of beds and the turnover of patients, moving patients through the continuum of care, managing appropriate length of stay, defining the scope of service, introducing technology, determining patient-staff ratios, and managing many other variables—all the while maintaining a safe environment, reducing pain and suffering, and improving satisfaction. Measurements can provide administrators with the infrastructure necessary to make informed decisions so that the organizational tightrope they walk becomes sturdier. Moreover, objective measures can promote improved communication with their governing bodies, their staffs, and their patients.

Hospital leadership has come a long way from a focus on balancing the budget and has moved away from considering the Joint Commission on Accreditation of Healthcare Organizations (JCAHO) surveys as inconvenient interruptions to the business-as-usual running of the organization. Because health care has changed, and because the social underpinnings of medical care have changed, health care professionals need to prepare themselves to meet these changes and not only to meet them but to greet them with an extended and welcoming hand.

The Joint Commission on Accreditation of Healthcare Organizations (JCAHO) is an independent, not-for-profit organization established more than fifty years ago to evaluate the quality and safety of care delivered by health care organizations. Its board of commissioners is made up of representatives of such nationally recognized professional organizations as the American Hospital Association, the American Medical Association, the American College of Physicians, the American Society of Internal Medicine, and the American College of Surgeons. JCAHO sets standards that measure health

care quality in the United States and around the world. For
a health care organization to be accredited, a team of JCAHO
health care professionals must do an extensive on-site review
of the organization's performance at least once every three
years. Accreditation is awarded based on how successfully
the organization meets JCAHO standards. Organizations are
evaluated through a review of their policies and procedures,
medical record reviews, performance improvement initiatives,
visits to patient care settings, interviews with staff and patients,
and staff competency evaluations.

Administrators mediate between the organization's governance
committees and the hospital employees, including the clinical staff. To
best do their job, administrators need experience in working with
quality measures in order to cope with the immense volume of statistical information related to their organization and to prioritize and
discriminate among different measures, as well as to use the information to set expectations for the staff. Administrators read financial reports with comfort, and they need to become comfortable with quality
reports in the same way. When they do, they will be able to help the
members of the board of trustees or other governance committees
evaluate services appropriately.

MEASURES AND MONEY

Administrators have always had to think about money, but today's
health care administrator needs to understand that profit is linked to
the quality of care being delivered. Years ago administrators did not
question clinical care; that was the exclusive purview of the physician.
And because physicians brought patients into the hospital and more
patients meant greater revenue for the hospital, administrators and
other health care managers were not eager to risk antagonizing physicians in any way by overseeing the way they treated their patients.

For many years reimbursement for services focused solely on the
volume of patients and the services given those patients. The issue was
always how much volume came in and what services were performed
rather than how successful the outcomes of that care were and what

the benefits to the patient were. If a patient had a long LOS and required surgery or additional support services, then Medicare reimbursed the hospital and the physicians for the number of days the patient was hospitalized and the services rendered.

Payment is related to the case mix index (CMI). Medicare introduced this classification system to encourage cost efficiencies in hospital care. Hospitals are paid a predetermined rate, depending on diagnosis and procedures required. Each Medicare patient is classified into a diagnosis related group (DRG), based on information from the medical record. The CMI is very useful in analysis because it reflects the relative severity of illness in a patient population. Surgery, for example, has a higher rate of reimbursement than most medical treatments have. Patient outcomes are not considered in determining case mix and payments. In fact hospitals can be paid more if a patient requires more surgery, even if it's due to a fall or an inappropriate initial treatment.

Today the major shaper of health care policy is the CMS, because that agency has been demanding answers to questions about quality of care and accountability for the delivery of services and because it provides the main economic force for hospitals and physicians. Today reimbursement depends not solely on volume but also on how good the delivered product is. Not all performance is equal, according to the CMS and JCAHO; payment and accreditation are related to good processes and outcomes. The way performance is evaluated is through objective measures. More than accreditation, meeting the CMS and JCAHO standards helps health care professionals to focus on improving operational and clinical processes.

The CMS evaluates hospitals and services on an ongoing basis and as moving targets. To increase reimbursement and to receive financial incentives the health care organization has to be in the top decile in the country in complying with quality indicators (such as giving aspirin to patients who come into the emergency department with AMIs). If one organization improves and another doesn't, then their respective rankings move accordingly up or down the scale. Profit is integrally connected to the measures that reveal quality of care. Therefore a good administrator needs to be familiar with quality indicators and with organizational processes associated with clinical care. Measures can identify areas of weakness in the delivery of care; measures can then monitor the improvements implemented; and measures can be used to correlate clinical, organizational, and financial performance.

MEASURES AND EVALUATING CARE

In years past, when defining a good hospital, no one considered accountability for the quality of care delivered. No one asked if the surgeries were successful or if the technological tests were appropriate or if there was efficient and effective use of resources. Only now are regulatory agencies and medical boards struggling with the concept of competence and privileging, a process that evaluates physician performance. Today these kinds of evaluations, which reveal quality, are reported and discussed in such public forums as newspapers and Web sites. Quality indicators, such as mortality rates, which had traditionally been discussed behind the closed doors of mortality and morbidity conferences or in medical journals or professional meetings, are now easily available to the public. Data open the door so that all can see what is happening at the bedside and demand accountability.

In today's health care climate, hospitals are watched and monitored as never before by regulatory and governmental agencies as well as the public. Therefore it behooves administrative leadership to learn how to use the processes of evaluation to improve care in the hospital. Objective information is a powerful weapon for reconciling the often conflicting agendas held by the organization, the medical staff, the regulatory and governmental agencies that monitor health care, and the patient. Today's administrators need to understand it all. They need to be able to define their product in order to sell it. Today's administrators need to know where the defects are in order to correct them.

If the physicians in your hospital are not giving beta-blockers or aspirin when the CMS standards say they should, leadership should know the reasons. If there is a serious event or an unexpected death, administrators need to know why it occurred and which processes should be improved to prevent a recurrence. Information is key, and not the subjective information that interprets medical care as an art form, understood by only a few well-credentialed and -schooled physicians. If a physician error results in patient harm, administrators need to understand what happened and be prepared to answer questions regarding services and maintaining safety. If patients are in danger, then the hospital, and the administrator, may have to face the consequences of dealing with the media and the community.

In addition to governmental agencies, private advocacy groups are also applying pressure on health care organizations to measure their care and monitor specific quality indicators. These groups also want proven value in return for their health care spending. Why shouldn't they? Health care used to be thought to be beyond the grasp of mere mortals, but no longer. Hospital administrators therefore have to be prepared to examine their organization's quality of care in the aggregate and use defined measurements to gather reliable data so they can prove that their organization is better than the competition.

What does it mean to be better? It means that when similar organizations are compared—with similar measures, risk adjusted to account for patient-specific information—one organization has a better ranking than another. Such rankings, which rely on compliance with evidence-based measures of quality, are being published as report cards and are available to the public so that patients can determine where they want to go for service and where they want their health care dollar to be spent. Patients taking on the role of informed consumers, industry and business organizations demanding specific services in return for their spending, and governmental and regulatory agencies focusing on quality indicators have created a revolution in the way health care is evaluated.

Through an understanding of process indicators (such as surgery) and outcome indicators (such as infection), the health care professional will become educated in the interrelationship of interventions and outcomes. For example, if a patient has to be readmitted after being discharged, it is important to analyze the reasons and to determine whether this event was due to a problem with technical skill, a lack of appropriate discharge planning, or random chance. With an understanding of measures, health care professionals will be better able to interpret data reports and then ask relevant questions. Through deliberate analysis an administrator can learn where to implement improvements or increase resources. Familiarity with quality management methodologies will promote accountability for quality care and enable leaders to meet the new challenges of the new health care competitive marketplace.

SUMMARY

To best manage their responsibilities, health care professionals should become familiar with the use of measurements to

- Evaluate the processes of care.
- Manage the interaction among physician, organizational, and patient needs and services.

- Balance the quality and cost of health care services.
- Promote accountability and improve communication among the professional and administrative staff.

Things to Think About

You are in a position to create and finance a hospital department.

- What questions would you want the answers to?
- Whom would you ask?
- What measures could you develop to get the answers to your questions?
- Why those measures and not others?
- How would you argue for or against this department to the governing body?
- What resources do you need (human, technological) to produce the best outcomes within a financially sound framework?
- What measure can you use to show that your service has an edge over the competition?

CHAPTER TWO

Fundamentals of Data

H ow do CEOs and senior leaders use data for decision making, and what data are available to them? These are important questions, because when leadership bases strategic, financial, and operational decisions on reliable data, the institution is managed well. When decisions are capricious and made without regard to facts, the institution suffers.

Too often leaders do not use data to drive decisions; rather, they formulate policy based on past experience, hire consultants to recommend changes, or allow reimbursement issues to dictate clinical, operational and financial decisions. Although data are available, leadership typically does not know how to use them for daily decision making or for developing long-range goals. In this chapter I will discuss the power of measures and databases to inform administrative, financial, and clinical decisions and the ways data can be used to influence changes and improvements in the delivery of care and the utilization of resources.

A good quality management process can help administrators understand clinical complications and explain the data. Data help leadership understand that, for example, patients who have hip replacements might also have the serious complication of a deep vein thrombosis (DVT, or blood clot). Without aggregated data there would be no way to recognize this significant problem. Without recognition, there is no possibility of improvement. Databases reveal trends. The quality management department supports these kinds of databases and analyses. Administrative leaders should see the value of using quality management data to understand and improve existing clinical practices and operational processes.

QUALITY AND FINANCE: A PERFECT FIT

Most administrative decisions are grounded on financial data. Financial data are developed by the chief financial officer (CFO) and the finance department. Financial decisions and strategic planning goals are built around controlling expenses. If financial indicators reveal that a hospital is not meeting its budget goals, then some expenses—and administrators generally determine which expenses—are trimmed. Although hospitals and health care institutions are centered on clinical services provided to patients, rarely, if ever, are clinical data integrated into the financial database. But they should be. It is important to the overall success of the hospital for its leadership to realize the fundamental relationship between financial and quality indicators.

Clinical data and information about organizational processes and procedures actually drive financial indicators. Yet for many administrators there is a disconnect between the clinical and financial reports; data about each are kept separate, and therefore they appear unrelated. However, with a moment's thought, connections become obvious. Reimbursement data and pay-for-performance incentives are based on diagnoses, treatment plans, physician orders, tests, length of stay (LOS), types of procedures, and resources required for care. Thus administrative data need to translate bedside care into economic variables that describe efficiency, appropriateness, and effectiveness of resource utilization, staff-patient ratios, or bed turnover rate. For malpractice data, risk and safety factors involved in care have to be understood.

Administrators are familiar with how to interpret financial data and how to make decisions by projecting from these data. Budgets are projections based on present or past financial data. Financial data are expected to be reliable and accurate, as the information is sent to external organizations and reimbursement is based on these data. When administrators become as comfortable with quality indicators as they are with financial data, they will be able to use that quality data to make informed predictions about the delivery of care, especially where problems may develop and where resources may be best employed.

Table 2.1 suggests how specific processes of care have either a positive or negative financial impact on the organization. Leadership should envision the hospital as a complex social organization with variables related to the process of care, their economic impact, and the positive and negative outcomes of interventions and treatment. For example, if a patient acquires an infection, the LOS is prolonged, and there may be no reimbursement if the LOS is longer than the benchmark set by the Centers for Medicare and Medicaid Services (CMS). Infection then costs the hospital money. If there is no infection, and the LOS is appropriate or short, it has a positive financial impact because the organization will be reimbursed and the bed can be used for another patient. Or consider a high-risk and expensive environment, such as the operating room. If a patient has to have a reoperation due to a complication, that has a negative financial impact because the operating room cannot be used for another patient and there may not be reimbursement for a repeat or repair of a procedure. Clearly, it makes good sense to consider quality-of-care variables in a financial statement. Defining expenses in terms of clinical outcomes, such as infection, provides leadership with information to evaluate staffing and other traditional expenses in the context of delivering quality care.

Using quality information to anticipate financial issues is most important. An administrator cannot look at the sources of reimburse-

	Cost Impact	
Process of Care	Positive	Negative
Hospital-wide nosocomial infection rate	No infection	Infection
	Short LOS	Long LOS
High-risk environment (cardiac surgery)	No complication	Complication
	Short LOS	Long LOS
Operating room	No complication	Reoperation
Intensive care unit	Minimal use	High consumption
Medication delivery	Minimal use	High consumption

Table 2.1. The Impact of Quality on Finance.

ment directly but can understand how revenue comes into the organization based on improved methods of care. Administrators can understand the budget through looking at processes of care; those processes are translated through measures into data.

The responsible health care leader learns to ask questions about the quality of care delivered to patients, and out of the answers to these questions, data arise, data that can be used for budgetary purposes. Not only should administrators know how to use the data available to ask intelligent questions and to ascertain problems, it is also important for them to know where these data are located and who is responsible for collecting and analyzing them and communicating information about them. Then, when it is necessary to make an informed decision (and when is it not?), the administrator knows whom to go to for reliable information.

QUALITY AND ACCOUNTABILITY

The quality management department collects data and should have analysts to develop databases (just as the finance department does) so that the organization's accountability for safe, quality care can be maintained. Too many administrators believe that quality management is about certification and regulatory compliance, and therefore limit the usefulness of that department. But the more information an administrator has about bedside care, the more involved he or she can be in the decisions about that care.

Realistically, it should be noted that clinicians may not always be eager to have administrators informed about care; they may have more autonomy when administrators don't understand clinical phenomena. However, because good outcomes, and quality care, are so crucial to the success, financial and otherwise, of the health care enterprise, health care professionals need to know as much as possible about the delivery of services that the hospital supplies. Without an understanding of clinical data—collected, analyzed, and provided by quality management—leadership is entirely dependent on physicians for an understanding and evaluation of care. And most physicians don't have a grasp of the whole picture, only their individual place in it. Quality management data have the advantage of being objective. Quality management has no agenda other than to monitor and assess care, whereas individual physicians treating specific patient populations may have a biased assessment of what is needed.

It is true that the Joint Commission on Accreditation of Healthcare Organizations (JCAHO), CMS, and other such agencies define the quality indicators health care organizations are expected to collect for evaluation and for accreditation. Unfortunately, too many administrators do not have knowledge of the broader importance of these data, and so they communicate that these data are valued only for their role in compliance. However, there are no better data to detail the progress of patient safety. Quality data, because they are mandated by accrediting agencies, are available but may in effect be lying on the floor, unused and unanalyzed.

When evidence, in the form of data, proves that good practices and good outcomes are being provided, reimbursement increases; patient advocacy groups, such as Leapfrog, invest their health care dollars for their employee health plans; and the media report good results, which serves to attract a greater number of patients to the hospital. When administrators realize that the variables they rely on to make decisions about operations and the budget are actually variables collected and analyzed for quality, their jobs are easier. They can determine factors about operational processes, information related to the clinical staff, elements associated with service quality, and variables related to resources, such as bed turnover and throughput.

The Leapfrog Group consists of over 170 companies and organizations that purchase health care for their employees. These companies are committed to reducing preventable medical mistakes and to improving the quality and affordability of health care services. They encourage the public reporting of quality indicators so that purchasing organizations and consumers can make more informed choices about which health care institution they should use. Because the group has vast economic power, it can dictate quality and safety standards for health care organizations. The group ranks hospitals throughout the country on promoting a culture of safety, communication among health care workers, communication between doctor and patient, success in preventing infections, level of medication errors, and level of complications.

Leaders who become informed through an understanding of quality data can participate in intelligent dialogues about problems and solutions. Few maverick CEOs and administrators are able to make the link among quality, financial, and clinical indicators and then move toward understanding interventions and levels of accountability. Successful leaders attempt to align quality and financial data and to understand clinical phenomena through data and measurements. Data connect administrative processes, clinical services, and finance.

LET THE WALLS COME TUMBLING DOWN

When administrative reports combine financial indicators, quality indicators, and clinical indicators in databases, organizational goals can be accurately represented. To establish such databases, it is necessary to define the clinical variables that actually shape the financial results of the hospital. Carrying out this definition process requires collaboration and communication among the finance department, quality management department, medical leadership, nursing leadership, and administration. The resulting data will provide leadership with a truer and clearer picture of what is occurring in their hospital, and accurate and objective information from the various departments will contribute to operational decisions.

However, this level of communication is not easy to achieve. How, for example, can a medical process be explained to a finance expert? For the medical expert the patient is a series of conditions that require interventions; for the finance expert the patient may be a source of revenue and the interventions expenses. Nurses have the responsibility of implementing both physician instructions and administrative expectations. Without objective data, these agendas lack coordination, and there is a risk that administrators will come to perceive the nurse as an expense rather than a person working "blind," without the right tools—data—to make decisions.

Using data to enhance collaboration among disciplines and departments across the organization has the further advantage of keeping the patient as the central focus. The quality management department establishes the clinical and operational variables that describe what happens at the bedside and in the workplace, from environmental and safety issues to clinical outcomes and process measures. The physician and the nursing staff supervise and enact clinical activities and oversee compliance with the rules and regulations that are imposed by external organizations, such as departments of health (DOHs) and JCAHO, and that focus on the patient and his or her care. Patient care dictates treatments and outcomes, which in turn influence financial variables, such as length of stay, particular environmental use, such as the ED or ICU, bed turnover, appropriate use of resources, and incidents.

When these data are combined, interrelationships among different parts of the organization are clearly revealed, and administrators and members of the board of trustees and other governance committees can garner information about the delivery of care. But this is in an ideal world and doesn't happen often. In reality even governance committees are divided along financial, clinical, and quality lines, and there is little exchange of information in board meetings. As a result, and in an attempt to avoid these distinctions and improve communication, JCAHO has recommended that board members receive information about quality.

FINDING ANSWERS

My voyage toward understanding the power and limitations of combining clinical data with financial and operational data for decision making began many years ago when the CEO of the health care system where I directed quality management activities came to the quality management office and asked me, "Is everything OK?" Just three words.

What was it that he really wanted to know? Because he knew his business and was very good at it, I knew that he wanted to know, at a minimum:

- If the length of stay for our patients was appropriate and we were not underusing or overusing our resources
- If our mortality rates were stable and low compared to the rates of other health systems, and if not, why not, and what we were doing to improve
- If bed turnover and wait times were efficient and reasonable
- If investments in various interventions and technologies were making a difference, both to patient health and safety and to the organization's financial equilibrium

- If there had been any adverse events or incidents requiring our ongoing monitoring for improvement
- If the hospitals in the system and the system as a whole were doing "better" this year than last

That one question, "Is everything OK?" contained all these other questions—and more.

Simply responding with, "Sure, things are great," would not have satisfied my CEO, or any other administrator who was looking to assess the performance of the organization. He wanted, expected, and deserved real answers, not sloppy, anecdotal, episodic, or personally subjective ones. His business background and experience had taught him that finance and quality were interdependent, and he wanted quality management to be integrated into every department of the hospital. More forward looking than most CEOs, he knew that regulatory organizations, such as JCAHO and the DOH, were using data and quality tools to enhance patient care and organizational performance. In order to answer his question properly, I needed to examine reliable, consistent data.

At most hospitals CEOs and senior administrators leave questions of a medical or clinical nature to the physicians, for several reasons. They feel that as nonclinicians they lack the necessary education to evaluate the clinical course of care. Also, administrators want to keep the physicians happy, because to a great extent the financial success of the hospital is dependent on the goodwill of the physicians, who bring their patients into the hospital. Physicians are not accustomed to being questioned by administrative staff. Their high level of technical competence as well as the length and intensity of their training make it difficult for physicians to be controlled by administration.

But because today's administrative leadership finds it increasingly necessary to understand measurements of quality and patient safety—such as mortality rates, infection rates, utilization rates, patient satisfaction rates, and much more—leaders also need to be able to understand and to evaluate care. To do so, they need data. As the organization's leaders, they are in charge and responsible; trustees, members of the community, and regulatory bodies ask them questions of a clinical nature and expect them to know the answers. Further, they are pressured by the government, the CMS, and the insurance companies to mediate between those who produce the hospital's product, the physicians, and those who pay for the treatment, the patients. Meeting these responsibilities is easier when objective data are available and used to analyze care.

OBJECTIFYING THE DELIVERY OF CARE

Determining the quality of care delivered to patients through data collection and analysis was spurred by JCAHO, which made data-driven processes a requirement for accreditation. For a health care organization to be accredited—and accreditation is accepted as the gold standard for the evaluation of care—data have to be the basis of actions taken and improvements monitored. One of the goals of using data to evaluate care has been to ensure that consistent standards are established and met for all organizations and that patient safety and quality care can be objectively assessed, measured, and improved. Standards are measured from zero compliance to full compliance.

What kinds of data are used, and where do they come from? Most CEOs and senior administrators don't have time to gather or analyze data; they hire staff to do it for them. Thus many administrators don't realize that they can elicit useful answers to important questions if they know how to use and interpret the data available to them. Figure 2.1 shows several databases available to administrators: some are internal to the organization; some are maintained by the states, and others by the federal government. When data are sitting in someone's computer unanalyzed and unprocessed, they won't do the administrator or anyone else any good. But when data are analyzed and interpreted, and these results are communicated effectively, these data can track and trend a wealth of information. Then leadership can use the data to intelligently assess and improve both clinical and organizational processes. The more data that are gathered and analyzed, the better the assessment will be.

Databases exist. For example, simple census data and administrative data, collected and trended over time by the state DOH, provide interesting information. Demographic data about patients reveal who is using the health care facilities, how old they are, what geographical areas they represent, what their primary and secondary diagnoses are, how long they stay in the hospital, what types of procedures or treatments they are given, what their discharge disposition is (home, nursing home) when they leave the hospital, and what kind of insurance they have.

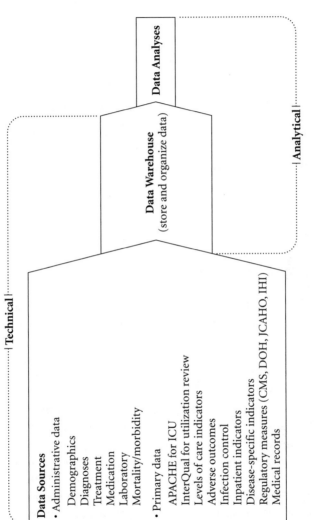

Data Sources
- Administrative data

  Demographics
  Diagnoses
  Treatment
  Medication
  Laboratory
  Mortality/morbidity

- Primary data

  APACHE for ICU
  InterQual for utilization review
  Levels of care indicators
  Adverse outcomes
  Infection control
  Inpatient indicators
  Disease-specific indicators
  Regulatory measures (CMS, DOH, JCAHO, IHI)
  Medical records

Data Warehouse
(store and organize data)

Data Analyses

|Technical|

|Analytical|

Figure 2.1. Quality Data Sources.

Information from these data could be used to address quality issues, such as rates of unexpected death or infection. Existing databases may require some reorganization before they can address specific questions, and therefore they may involve administrative investment. If the senior leadership wants to better understand the delivery of services, including clinical services, in the organization, it will invest in database development. Data development should conform to the questions that administrators are interested in answering.

CASE EXAMPLE: CARDIAC MORTALITY

Here's an example of how data can influence the provision of care. Several years ago New York State published information about mortality rates for cardiac surgery. In the health care system where I work, we learned from these data that one of our flagship hospitals had a higher cardiac surgery mortality rate than the comparable hospitals in our region. The media were all over this news, and the CEO, as well as members of the board of trustees, wanted to know what was going on. The medical staff gave the expected responses, that their patients were high risk or that other institutions didn't accept such sick patients for fear of having a high mortality rate reported. That answer was accepted—the first year. Typically, when this kind of bad publicity appears, senior administrators start changing medical staff, but unless the problem is one of clinical competency, getting rid of staff, or reengineering, doesn't address the issue. It is much more effective to analyze information in order to arrive at a solution; therefore when the same results were published a second year, the CEO empowered the quality management department to analyze the situation.

The mortality data collected and reported by the New York State DOH introduced several very important ideas to our data formulation: definitions of risk adjustment, expected outcome, and benchmarking. Risk adjustment involves a complex formula designed to account for differences among the patient population and to ensure valid comparisons. With these concepts, performance across hospitals can be measured and compared, apples to apples, so to speak. Statistical analysis of the high-risk population at issue enabled me and my staff to compare the cardiac care provided by our institution with that of other institutions in the light of a rational science, rather than from the viewpoint of emotion or the prestige of the physicians. Note also that the efforts made to reduce mortality were spurred by external sources, data from the state DOH and pressure from the media, and not by sources internal to the hospital.

> Risk adjustment refers to a statistical process that is used to identify and adjust for variation among patients, especially for those characteristics that have an impact on patient outcomes. Owing to these varying characteristics or risk factors, patients can experience different outcomes, regardless of the quality of care provided. Applying a formula that accounts for differences allows comparisons of patient outcomes across organizations that are fair and accurate.

To effectively change clinical practices, quality management data should be supplied in a manner that evokes respect from the medical staff. For example, to overcome the notion that patients are sicker and have more complicated conditions at one institution than at another, quality analysts should be sure to use risk-adjusted data. Once risk-adjusted data level the playing field among different hospitals (or units within a hospital), one can look at patient-specific data to discover causes of variation from the standard of care. In our system, quality management staff examined the available administrative data; this information revealed that the high mortality rate for our cardiac patients was associated with a secondary diagnosis of sternal wound infection or sepsis.

The data also showed that cardiac patients had cardiac surgery at different levels of urgency: emergency, urgent, or elective (that is, planned). Information about the age, gender, and LOS of these patients was also available. So what? How do these pieces of information help solve the mystery of what was going wrong? Establishing the answer may not immediately solve the problem but will identify areas that should be targeted for change.

Data analysis showed that those patients who had emergency surgery were readmitted to the operating room (OR) for bleeding more frequently than other patients. These unplanned readmissions and reoperations resulted in prolonged hospital stays, which in turn increased the risk and the incidence of wound infections. In other words, those patients who had emergency surgery, had bleeding, and were readmitted for treatment were the ones who were dying from sepsis at a higher rate than other patients.

At this point I wanted to understand what was causing the bleeding, and why this particular group, the emergency patients, were the most vulnerable. Further data detective work revealed a process difference between this group and the other cardiac patients. One preoperative process for cardiac surgery patients is to stop taking anticoagulants, such as blood thinners like aspirin, for a set period of time. Because emergency patients had little or no forewarning of their surgery, they hadn't stopped this medication and therefore had greater incidences of complications from bleeding. Once the data helped to identify the source of the problem, preventive steps could be taken, such as giving these patients clotting medication after surgery.

Within two years after we had used data to understand this delivery of care, the DOH data reported that our hospital now had the lowest mortality rate in the state—that it was the "best." Everyone involved in treating cardiac surgery patients was pleased to have the information and to understand the causality of the problems. Excellence in care is measurable through such indicators as mortality, infection, LOS, unplanned readmissions, self-extubation rates (patients removing their own ventilator tubes), informed consent, and so on. These variables—all quality indicators—can be defined, tracked, and trended over time. The data analysis also resulted in the formulation of new policies by the physicians, who clarified the expected standard of care for their patients and increased oversight of physician competence. Everyone benefited.

CASE EXAMPLE: INTENSIVE CARE UNITS

Another way in which data analysis can make an impact on patient care and organizational processes was brought home to me through intensive care unit (ICU) care and expenditure issues. An ICU is highly resource intensive, both of staff and technology, because the patients served generally have multiple serious health problems that require many services. At a meeting of our system's senior staff several years ago, the finance officer announced that the expense of operating the ICUs was creating an unstable financial environment for the system, and he made the suggestion that something be done to curb expenses.

Administrators responsible for these kinds of decisions have to be very cautious when considering reducing services and resources, to ensure that there is no negative impact on patient safety. Physicians may argue against any ICU cuts as well, because they generally believe that their patients require ICU care. My staff and I suspected that patients were being admitted into the ICUs according to poorly defined criteria, which meant that resources were not being used appropriately.

Data revealed that the ICU patients had a great deal of variability in severity of illness. Some patients were there for observation or were in stable condition waiting for lab results; some were there for end-of-life care; some needed intensive care resources. There was no individual who was accountable for the patient population; no one was in charge. There was no gatekeeper for this most complex unit of the hospital. Physicians did not want to monitor or second-guess their colleagues and suggest that some patients be in other units. But the lack of clear admission criteria created bottlenecks in patient throughput, and in some cases, when patients in the ED or in postoperative recovery units had to wait for an ICU bed to become available, LOS was extended unnecessarily. For administration, improving ICU admission criteria would improve efficiency and help to manage patient flow, but making suggestions might antagonize physicians, who might feel that their clinical judgment was being questioned.

The best way to manage such somewhat opposing forces is to introduce objective science and deliberate methods. After doing extensive research the quality management staff recommended to the CEO that the health system purchase a critical care patient screening tool called APACHE (Acute Physiology, Age and Chronic Health Evaluation). This objective scale records the patient population, case mix, length of stay, severity of illness, and levels of care required for critically ill adults. Even hospital mortality is assessed through a severity score and a predictive equation. With this tool, objective and clearly defined data would drive decision making and strategic planning for quality care of critically ill patients. However, some medical staff were concerned that the tool would override their clinical judgment and objected to the time and effort involved in data entry and analyses.

Administrators, who had been looking to streamline the ICUs and improve their efficiency, supported the APACHE methodology. Many physicians became supportive because the data gave them an opportunity to measure their own performance and evaluate their processes and procedures. Table 2.2 shows the indicators in the database used to monitor ICU care in our health system hospitals. By comparing the data of different variables over time, such as LOS, mortalities, and readmissions to the unit, leadership was able to accurately assess the

Indicators	2003	2004	2005
Number of discharges			
Number of admissions			
Number of low-risk patients (based on APACHE score)			
ICU LOS			
Number of mortalities			
Number of self-extubations			
Number of ventilated patients			
Number of readmissions within 72 hours			
Number of do-not-resuscitate (DNR) patients			

Table 2.2. Intensive Care Unit Data Collected by System Hospitals.

delivery of care and determine where improvement efforts should be targeted.

Data became a vehicle for illustrating that the standard of care in the ICUs was appropriate and that patients were being effectively treated. Data also spurred communication among physicians about care and its consequences. Improvement could be reported at upper-level performance improvement committees, with concrete data as support for assertions of success. However, it took an evaluative methodology that reviewed each case to convince physicians that the measure was intended to enhance their clinical judgment, not override it.

DEFINING GOALS

Leadership support and organizational commitment are required for collecting and analyzing reliable data, whether financial, quality, or operational. Senior administrators have to define for themselves and their staff the level of excellence, or quality, of the organization they want to lead. Commitment to data and commitment to a quality organization go hand in hand. For example, when the Institute of Medicine and other medical agencies report that people are dying unnecessarily in hospitals due to infection, it behooves the hospital administrator who wants to run an excellent institution to inquire into the infection rates at his or her hospital in order to identify any problem that should be monitored.

Yet most institutions don't monitor their infection rate, and those that do say that their infection rate is very low. If that were true, it is hard to see why infection is the major variable associated with death of hospitalized patients in the United States. Clearly organizations are not monitoring or measuring or reporting their rates of infection accurately. They are using the ostrich approach to information: don't ask, don't tell. However, poor care usually has a way of making itself known—to the patients and to the public—typically through an event that comes to the attention of the news media.

Administrators who value patient safety and want to run an excellent health care institution should develop a database for prevention and should monitor infection rates and hold staff accountable for ensuring that the rates are low. Data can be used to ascertain where the gaps exist in providing safe patient care. Data reveal whether the infection is contained in a specific area or unit of the hospital or is related to specific staff or involves engineering or materials.

NOTHING NEW UNDER THE SUN

Recent media attention has brought to public view an increasing incidence of infection. For example, the media in England have focused on MRSA. MRSA stands for methicillin-resistant *Staphylococcus aureus,* but the term is now used as shorthand for any strain of staph bacteria resistant to antibiotics. Hospitalized patients who contract MRSA are at risk for serious infection and pneumonia.

Most infections are caused by the age-old problem of poor hygiene—especially caregivers' failure to wash their hands appropriately. No high-tech solutions are required to fix the problem, no extraordinary financial outlay; nonetheless, in many organizations it remains an intractable problem. So much so that the British Parliament made the suggestion that patients should remind their physicians to wash their hands, but patient advocacy groups protested that that would impose too much responsibility on patients, who may feel reluctant or be unable to police their physicians.

Difficulties with hand washing have been blamed on having too few sinks or sinks inappropriately placed. When organizations install more sinks and expect to reduce infection, it doesn't work; infection remains high and hand washing remains the source of the problem.

One hospital, hoping to reduce its infection rate, even tried assigning a nurse in the ICUs to "watch" each physician who left a patient's room and to remind that physician to wash his or her hands between patients. Florence Nightingale, I am sure, is turning over in her grave. Until quality care is internalized by every decision maker and every member of the organization and patient safety is regarded as paramount, interventions will function like little Band-Aids rather than fundamentally improved processes. Using measures to assess, monitor, and evaluate care helps to convince staff that there is an ongoing problem that requires improved education or new processes.

CASE EXAMPLE: FALLS

Using data to improve patient safety is not only required by governmental agencies but has become a recent focus of media attention. The reason regulatory agencies require data about falls, for example, is that falls are prioritized as a high-risk problem that can result in fractures, surgery, or worse. Because falls are a patient safety concern, if safety is a high priority for the organization, part of its stated mission, then preventing falls is important.

Nursing staff collect information about falls: incident reports record the time, place, date, frequency, and reason for the fall. Patient assessment and H&P (history and physical) target certain patients as highly susceptible to falling. Falls have an impact on LOS, especially when the resulting injuries require tests and treatment. Patients who fall, and their families, complain about their care in a formal way, such as through satisfaction surveys or complaints to the organization, suggesting that better care would have prevented the fall from occurring. Patients and their families have instituted lawsuits as a result of falls.

Malpractice suits are increasingly being brought after falls, because they are thought to be preventable and can result in serious injury. Jury awards for these perceived "unnecessary" complications have been high. Why is it that hospitals cannot prevent patient falls? The methodological explanation is that the "fall prevention" ranking (that is, a given patient's likelihood of falling) is perceived to be a nursing assessment issue. This perception is itself a problem, due to the conflicting desires to show not only that the rates are low but also to illustrate to regulatory agencies that the measure, which they require, is being used. In fact, the report of low rates is based on poorly defined measures.

A valid measure defines a set of events that occurs in a circumstance where there were opportunities for that type of event to occur.

Figure 2.2 graphically illustrates how to define a quality measure. The number of events is the *numerator* of the measure, and the number of opportunities for that event to occur is the *denominator*.

For example, if you are interested in examining how many falls resulted in fractures, the numerator of the measure would be exactly that—the number of patient falls that resulted in fractures. The denominator would encompass the totality of all falls. If 20 falls resulted in fractures, and there were 100 falls in total, the numerator (20) is a subset of the denominator (100). The measure of the falls is calculated as a rate, in this case, 20/100, or 20 percent. The numerator, or N of a measure, defines what you want to study or what question you want to investigate or which hypothesis you want to test. Therefore the N can be as specific or as general as appropriate. If you were interested in determining the influence of medication on falls, you might want to know the rate of medicated patients who fell. The measure would be events/opportunities, or N/D—in this case the number of patients on sedatives who fell/the total number of patients who fell (see Figure 2.3).

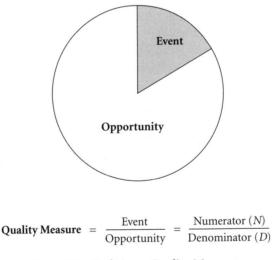

$$\textbf{Quality Measure} \ = \ \frac{\text{Event}}{\text{Opportunity}} \ = \ \frac{\text{Numerator } (N)}{\text{Denominator } (D)}$$

Figure 2.2. Defining a Quality Measure.

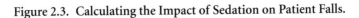

$$\frac{\text{Event}}{\text{Opportunity}} = \frac{N}{D} = \frac{\text{Number of Sedated Patients Who Fell}}{\text{Total Number of Patient Falls}}$$

Figure 2.3. Calculating the Impact of Sedation on Patient Falls.

Because major falls that cause injury and even death still occur, the focus is shifting from reacting to an event toward developing prevention programs. Another reason to adopt such a focus is that the majority of today's hospital patient population is at high risk for falls because they are increasingly elderly, living longer, experiencing multiple diseases, and taking many medications. Even those organizations that have developed a falls prevention program have a high rate of falls because the assessment and program can be so routinized that it becomes a paper exercise to illustrate to the accreditation agencies that the organization is in compliance with assessing patients.

There are organizations that believe if there are no falls being reported, there are no falls occurring. Patent nonsense. The New York State Commissioner of Health has taken an extremely hard-line approach to the reporting of errors and is critical of hospitals that underreport. She is quite right to take this position, because without information, improvements cannot be intelligently implemented.

In our health care system it took almost eight months to develop a definition of "fall" that was acceptable to all caregivers. What might seem to a layperson a straightforward concept can be quite complicated. For example, does a "fall" have to result in the patient being on the floor? Can a patient "fall" if that patient is being assisted onto a chair by a caregiver? Does a "fall" have to be observed by another to distinguish it from a collapse or a faint? Measurements cannot be standardized unless everyone involved in data collection understands what data they are collecting.

It's obvious that if the reasons for the falls are understood and if appropriate improvements can be developed and implemented, that would decrease the incidence of falls. This decrease would produce many advantages: the organization's safety objectives would be met, the potential for malpractice claims against the hospital would be reduced, patient satisfaction would be increased, the budget would no longer be adversely affected by costs of falls, LOS would be reduced, and most important, patient safety would be preserved.

With data, professionals can understand the scope of the problem they have and determine whether resources should be used for improvements. If you have 10 falls per 1,000 patients (1 percent), over the course of six months, perhaps you would determine that your improvement efforts should be focused elsewhere. But if you discover that your unit or hospital has 10 falls per 50 patients, or 20 percent every week, you know you have a far more serious problem to address.

You need a sense of the dimensions of the problem, that is, data that reveal how many incidents (the numerator of the measure) were related to how many possibilities (the denominator), and also a time frame to delimit that data, to help you measure, or quantify, the incidence of falls, or any other variable. The numerator of a measure is defined by the question being considered, such as do elderly patients with diabetes have an increased likelihood of a fall? With data, such questions can be answered accurately.

Data can be gathered on patient age, patient diagnosis, and the time when (on what shift) the patient falls. In addition, information is readily available on the patient-staff ratio at the time of the fall, on the unit of the patient who falls, and on the cause of the fall. There can be many variables to assess. Was the call bell not answered in a timely way? Was there an obstruction on the floor? Were the lights not working properly? Did medication play a part? What happened to the patient is also documented: was there an injury, what kind of injury was it, what was the cost in terms of LOS, and what were the unanticipated services (return to the OR) or clinical outcomes, such as infection or malpractice suits? All these pieces of data are associated with measures. Taken together the information enables an administrator to grasp the situation in a complex way (rather than to assume the nurse was not doing her or his job) and implement improvements. Good administrators have valid data underlying their decisions. Data collection and analyses should also be the responsibility of clinical supervisors, such as the head nurses and the chairs of clinical departments.

Regulatory agencies require hospitals and health care organizations to correlate human resource indicators, such as staffing ratios, with quality indicators, such as falls. A common suggestion that makes a kind of intuitive sense is that patient falls are related to the number of nurses and other health care staff available for bedside care on the unit, if deployed appropriately. However, in our system, when we collected information that tracked staffing turnover with the rate of falls (see Figure 2.4), it appeared there was no correlation between them. Our conclusion was that a single indicator (that is, staffing) was insufficient to explain as complex a phenomenon as falls. For example, case mix index, that is the degree of illness associated with specific diagnoses, in combination with staffing ratios, may be more informative about patients at risk for falls. Without these data, leadership might have been tempted to increase staff, with the associated expense, to reduce falls—without success.

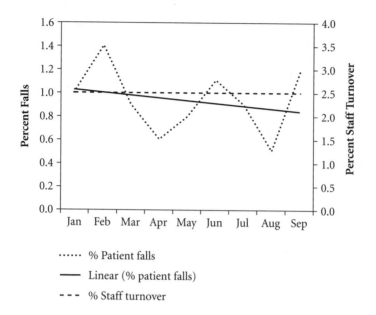

Figure 2.4. Patient Falls and Staff Turnover, January–September.

COMMUNICATING INFORMATION FROM QUALITY MEASURES

Once analyzed, data need to be communicated appropriately and to the appropriate people. Quality management staff can assist administrators with methods of data presentation that are effective for different venues and specific audiences, whether clinical groups, such as the medical boards, or institutional governance or administrative groups, or governmental audiences for accreditation.

Data can be presented in various ways, again depending on what is being presented and to what audience. Let's assume a high-level administrative committee is interested in understanding patient falls because this is a safety issue. So people can understand the kind of improvements that need to be made, data can be gathered on various variables. One such variable is time of occurrence.

Figure 2.5 reveals, through a simple pie chart, that in the unit investigated more falls occur during the night than at any other time. This information makes intuitive sense, but having the data to support an impression concretizes the problem and also sets a baseline against which to measure improvement efforts. Once you have this informa-

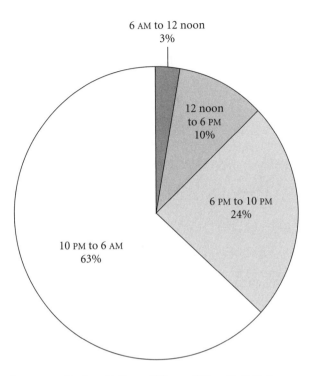

Figure 2.5. Patient Falls and Time of Day, Unit X, January.

tion, you can investigate why falls occur at night. It may be due to limited visibility, poor lighting, the staff ratio, or patient disorientation.

Depending on what you want to know, you can drill down to highly specific levels, such as examining data by day of the week for a single unit (or units). Figure 2.6 shows, by means of a simple run chart, that the fall rate on the unit investigated is highest on weekends and especially on Saturday. Improving staffing ratios or staff education might improve this situation. However, it doesn't make sense to spend money hoping to solve a problem before you understand its dimensions.

It may also be of interest to senior staff to discover the relationship between the falls rate and patients with specific diagnoses. Therefore data can also be collected according to diagnosis. Figure 2.7 shows, by means of a simple bar chart, that on the unit investigated patients with diabetes fall at a greater rate than others. Education can then be targeted at this group of patients and at their caregivers in order to effect changed practices.

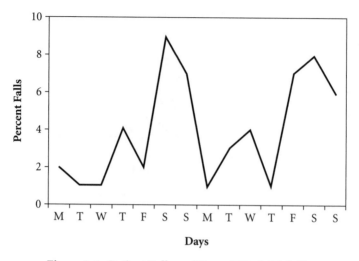

Figure 2.6. Patient Falls and Day of Week, Unit X.

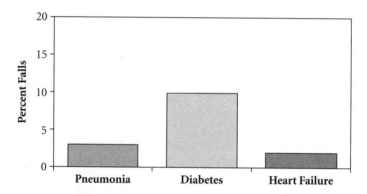

Figure 2.7. Patient Falls and Three Disease Conditions, Unit X.

Depending on the parameters of the analysis, data reveal different issues, which can be displayed in different graphic formats, according to what works best. Once the data have illuminated problem areas, resources can be invested in improvements. Measuring services on a continuous basis over time also allows trends to be observed. Because pieces of information are simply that—disconnected pieces—you need to collect data over time in order to observe patterns.

LEADERSHIP DEFINES
THE LEVEL OF QUALITY

Leadership sets the tone for the entire organization, including the attitude people in the organization will adopt toward defining quality measures, collecting data, analyzing the data, and communicating the results. Measurements must be performed carefully; be an essential part of performance improvement efforts; be put before the medical boards, the trustees, and the administration; and be the basis of all patient safety initiatives.

For example, the incidence and severity of pressure injuries, or decubiti (what used to be called bedsores) have been monitored for decades because this painful and potentially dangerous condition is entirely preventable. Yet today the government is still forced to mandate that health care organizations take steps to reduce the incidence and severity of pressure injuries. It is not rocket science to turn immobilized bedridden patients so that their skin retains its integrity and is not vulnerable to painful irritation and infection. Wouldn't a CEO or senior administrator want to know if the hospital's rate of pressure injuries is high and, if so, why it is high—and not because the government tells the hospital to monitor this rate but because the CEO or administrator is committed to heading an institution that can pride itself on delivering good care?

Traditional safety issues can be monitored and understood through objective measurements collected over time. There are national benchmarks for, for example, pressure injuries. If data concerning the volume and severity of pressure injuries are reliably collected and analyzed, an administrator can question why certain units are performing below the standard. Also, an administrator can gain information about the connection between pressure injuries and extended LOS. It is an empirical question whether patients who acquire a pressure injury stay longer in the hospital, require increased treatments, have infections, or tend to have certain diseases. There is no mystery underlying these questions. Measurements can provide answers.

Improving care requires leadership commitment to an issue. If clinicians tell an administrator not to worry about pressure injuries, that it's not a big problem or that the rate is acceptable and normal, and if the administrator doesn't ask for the objective data and insist on seeing improvements, the message that is communicated is that the administrator doesn't really want to monitor care. But if the administrator asks the quality management department to define a pressure injury measure so that data can be collected that are uniform and reliable, or even better, do what we do in our system, which is to use an objective scale, collect data on incidence and severity, and report those data monthly, and if the administrator insists on seeing improvements through these data, then the organization gets a different message. Staff are going to be held accountable by the leadership for the delivery of good care on an ongoing basis.

FINDING QUESTIONS

Collecting and monitoring data can be thought of as fishing: depending on what you want to catch, that's how wide you throw your net. If you want only a specific bit of information, you tailor your measure so that you collect that information and no other. For example, you might want to know how many patients from a specific nursing home enter the hospital with preexisting pressure injuries, or you might want information about the prevalence of pressure injuries among elderly diabetic patients. Measures can be global or highly specific. Just as *Consumer Reports* helps purchasers determine what car or washing machine they should buy by rating models according to the specific qualities they are looking for, quality measures of health care services can evaluate the specifics of various services.

When there are problems (and there always are!), a responsible administrator has to manage them. An administrator would not go to the CEO and say there is "some kind of problem" in dialysis and that the state inspector has found the water used was not cultured (tested for pathogens) and therefore might not have been clean and might be a source of infection. If the administrator has developed a process that provides constant measurement of the sterility of the water, such a problem could not occur. If such a problem does occur, there has to be an effort to change practices and overhaul the procedures used and improve them. Again, the administrator is at the head and has to lead the charge by investing in the process. Change is always difficult to introduce, and buy-in from professional staff has to be courted. Education has to be implemented. Above all, the changed process needs to be measured and evaluated constantly and consistently to determine what impact the improvement is making.

Or take another example. If a behavioral unit or hospital has a high elopement rate (that is, patients leaving without authorization) and an increased incidence of suicide, how do you investigate the processes involved? Is the door to the roof left open? Who is accountable for maintaining security? Are there other environmental factors involved, or is the problem related to medication, or are there staffing competency issues? How does an administrator know the answer to such questions?

Collecting reliable data allows those responsible for the safety of patients to promote best practices and positive outcomes. Without data, we are all walking around not only in the dark but blindfolded.

SUMMARY

Health care leaders should use data and develop measures and databases in order to

- Assess, monitor, and improve the delivery of care.
- Understand the relationship among clinical, financial, and operational processes.
- Mediate between those who deliver care (the physicians) and those who pay for that care (the patients and the insurance companies).
- Monitor care in accordance with JCAHO and CMS regulations.
- Communicate information about aggregated data in order to change physician practices.
- Identify areas for improvement in the delivery of care.
- Support strategic planning.
- Derive answers to questions.
- Determine where best to invest resources.

Things to Think About

A patient satisfaction survey has reported that patients are leaving the emergency department at your hospital without being seen and have complained about the ED to the media. The CEO has asked you to investigate.

- How would you determine the cause of the problem?
- How would you determine the extent of the problem?

- How would you evaluate the impact of the problem on patient safety? On the organization?
- Whom would you work with to improve the situation?
- How would you conclude that improvements have been made?
- What data would you use?
- Where would you get these data?
- How would you evaluate the cost of the improvements in relation to the benefit?

CHAPTER THREE

Using Data to Improve Organizational Processes

uriously, unlike other kinds of business organizations, health care institutions don't generally make use of quality data and measurements to improve their profit margins and enhance their organizational performance. It would be unthinkable for the leaders of Toyota or Wal-Mart, for example, to ignore data that could reveal problems or opportunities for improvement; yet health care leaders frequently ignore information revealed in data that are readily available to them.

The link between quality and finance is clear when leadership realizes that promoting successful patient outcomes can improve market share and the efficient use of resources while decreasing unnecessary expenditures. Data about quality can be used to develop effective criteria for resource allocation and improvement efforts, to promote accountability, and to improve communication with staff. In this chapter I will suggest ways in which organizations can establish a culture of quality and overcome traditional resistance to using measures to quantify health care practices; I will also explain how analyzing data can lead to organizational, clinical, and financial improvements.

SATISFYING THE
DEMANDING CONSUMER

If health care is viewed as composed of products, parallel in many re-
spects to automobiles or refrigerators, traditional ideas about how to
manage hospitals become obsolete. Think of the hospital as supplying a consumer of health care with such specific products as wound
care, cardiac services, oncological services, behavioral health services,
and so forth. Consumers of these products are either satisfied or not.
If they are satisfied, the hospital is successful because patients return
when they need more products and they also recommend the quality
of care and excellence of services to others. In addition, physicians
want to be associated with successful organizations. Simple syllogisms,
perhaps, but I am trying to make a point.

Evidence-based medicine (EBM) is a paradigm for evaluating
health care services through research, such as randomized
controlled trials, and through expert analyses of algorithms
of care. The dissemination of information is also emphasized
in EBM, in order for the evidence to reach clinical practice or
for the results of research to reach the bedside. Generally, EBM
integrates the most comprehensive and up-to-date research
with clinical expertise.

It is important for those involved in hospital organization and administration to internalize the values of evidence-based medicine as
more than an act of compliance; it is the right thing to do. If a patient
has had a hip surgery and doesn't feel well, and if his or her vital signs
suggest infection, sometimes clinicians wait before doing tests or making an intervention. In contrast, when using guidelines that are derived from EBM, care is proactive, so that the caregiver checks whether
the antibiotic protocol was followed—that is, was the correct antibiotic administered at the right time and discontinued appropriately.
EBM provides an outline for the standard of care.

In the same way, a measure reflects good care. For example, when a
patient's vital signs are stabilized at a certain level, that information
can be among the criteria for discharge from the recovery room to the
floor unit. Without measures or guidelines individual physicians can

react in a variety of ways; with guidelines and measures there is less variation in treatment protocols because interventions are clearly indicated and expected. Again, measures are more than an indicator of compliance with regulatory recommendations; they are useful for studying, analyzing, and improving care delivery. A measure can be developed to monitor how many patients who received a specific treatment or who had the same procedure had successful outcomes, and if not, data can provide information about why not.

Today's patients do their homework and know what to expect. Patients know they are the buyers of health care services, and they feel within their rights to demand a totality of good care, not just scattered bits and pieces. The combination of patients as consumers and guidelines for appropriate treatment is redefining health care as a product that can be purchased and evaluated like many others. The media have been quick to understand how to evaluate the product through measures, quicker than the medical establishment. Hospitals are ranked and classified accordingly.

OFFERING VALUE

Once this idea of health care services as a product is accepted, the challenge is to define *value* for that product. A business organization offers its customers value by carefully defining a standard for its product. Compare buying health care services and buying a car. If you have the means to buy any car you choose, you can buy a sports car because you like its looks and enjoy its speed, or for a similar price, you can buy a sedan because you value the safety and comfort of its ride (see Figure 3.1).

In other words, your expectations and your personal requirements dictate the car's value—to you. There is no single standard for providing value to all consumers; the value is dependent on the consumer's expectations. Health care value can be considered along the same lines. However, poor value is obvious. Just as no one wants to purchase a car that breaks down while pulling away from the sales lot, no one wants to die in a hospital because of a medical error. Compliance with evidence-based measures is a minimal expectation for a standard of care.

One of the reasons the cost of health care is increasing astronomically is that most senior leaders don't understand this idea of providing customers with value. Some leaders think that hiring more staff

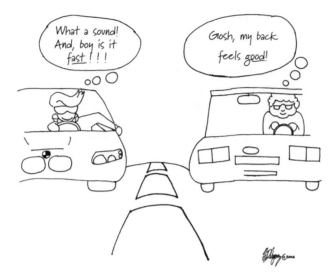

Figure 3.1. What Is Important to You?

to ensure compliance with measures will provide value, but what they are doing is multiplying the expense of care without increasing the value of that care. It would be much better for all involved, patients and organizational leadership, to instill the value of good care, to understand that providing good care is good business, and to encourage the idea that evidence-based medicine practices help clinical staff to avoid unnecessary variations in care. If an institution can show compliance with recommended measures, it may seem on the surface as if it is delivering good value to its customers. But when a hospital's leaders are simply trying to fill out the right forms to ensure government reimbursement, customers will not be satisfied, and eventually the care will be shown to be inadequate.

Here's another way to think of this issue: Which is the better hospital, one that is ranked in the top decile in the country according to CMS (Centers for Medicare and Medicaid Services) measures and that requires minimal resources because good care is integrated into the fabric of the organization, or one that achieves the top decile due to employing many case managers and using software to ensure that its documentation is accurate. The rankings and the measures should be viewed—again, by both patients and leadership—not as an end in themselves but as representing a concept that describes a clinical phenomenon. If physicians in the emergency department (ED) are not administering aspirin to patients arriving with acute myocardial infarction (AMI)—as EBM says they should and as the CMS dictates—why not? From my point of view, unnecessary variation, by which I mean variation from the standard, is the same as a defect in care.

SHOWING THE NUMBERS

If leadership wants to understand what is going on in the organization, rather than ask for subjective opinions from clinicians and others who may have vested interests in or limited exposure to the processes involved in various arenas in the hospital, leaders should use numbers to quantify the phenomenon or problem. Numbers can usually quantify even extremely abstract concepts. For example, years ago, when patients were in pain, physicians and staff recognized their pain from their expressions and gestures or because they complained. However, pain was thought to be so amorphous and so personal that it could not be measured. But it can be, and now it is. Regulatory agencies mandate not only that pain be measured but that it be controlled and measured over time for improvement. Physicians are required to prescribe medication to maintain the comfort of the patient. Pain management is defined as a patient's right. Reducing and controlling pain is more than simply humane. Evidence shows that pain relief contributes to patient recovery, increased mobility, and an improved level of functioning.

Many abstract or relative concepts can be measured. We are a culture of number-conscious consumers. We go to five-star restaurants and buy top-ranked computers. If you are the manager of a bank and your customers complain because they wait "too long" in line, how can you understand the meaning of *too long* or even *long?* You can determine a value for *long*, even an arbitrary one—say, if five people are on a line they will have too long a wait. And then you count over time, at regular intervals, how long the lines are. At the times when there are often five people waiting on line, perhaps you will want to rethink the staffing of the windows. Simply assigning the idea of *long* to the number five is useful for analysis and useful for your staff as well. If they know that lines with over five people are considered a problem, they have an objective reality for the notion of *long*.

The same is true with pain. Pain level can be determined through a scale and assigned a value (see Figure 3.2). Following medical

How much pain are you in?

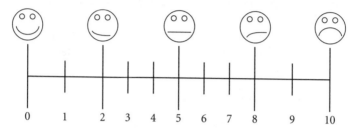

Figure 3.2. Pain Assessment Scale.

intervention, pain can be remeasured, thereby evaluating the success of the intervention. If the intervention is not successful, medication can be further adjusted, and then the pain can be remeasured. Because pain is subjective to the patient, the patient is the only person who can evaluate the success of the medication. Without an objective measure, everyone is floundering around without information.

MEASURES ARE GOOD BUSINESS

Providing health care is a service, and hospitals are businesses that must be financially viable to survive. Therefore, having the capacity to assess the components of its business is critical to a hospital's success. We can use any business as an example to understand the value of objective assessment and its relation to improved success. Imagine that you manage a hospital's food or nutrition department (or that you own a pizza parlor), and you want to improve your service (or increase your profits). How would you go about it? You would probably start out by counting your volume, which would provide you with a baseline, and then you would include special dietary needs (or special orders). Once you know the scope of the services provided, you will be able to make comparisons over time and to predict the volume of trays, workload, and turnaround time. What makes a successful food delivery program, or what indicators make an impact on clinical outcomes and patient satisfaction? You can think about this, talk to nurses and physicians (or other pizza parlor owners), and read the available literature about your service, and that way you might collect a list of ideas about success.

Some indicators might reflect the delivery service: is the right order delivered at the right temperature to the right patient (customer) in a timely way? That's four indicators: correctness of order, temperature on delivery, correctness of bed (address), and timeliness. Each of these indicators can be measured over time. If the collected data reveal a problem in one or more of these areas, you could focus your efforts on improving that area. Unless you know what to fix, you can't make improvements.

You might not stop there. Because you are in the business of providing a service, you might also be concerned about consumer satisfaction. You might decide to include a questionnaire about patient satisfaction with the food delivery and then to assess from patient responses areas where improvements should be made.

It is also productive in a medical service, or any other consumer business, to assess staff competency. Are the staff well trained? Do they have a sense of loyalty and commitment to the work or the organization? What is the staff turnover rate and what are some of the reasons for staff turnover? If your goal is to increase profitability, data may reveal a link between a competent and loyal workforce and increased efficiency.

As a manager, you would collect information about all these indicators and monitor them over time in order to develop a sense of the service and also to see if there are relationships among any of the indicators. After you learn about issues, you can begin to develop appropriate improvements and put resources to good use. Say you determine that staff turnover is an issue because allowing time for training is not cost effective. How can you improve the situation? What kind of education would be appropriate for your staff? Is there an incentive program you might introduce to keep staff happy longer? The quality methodology of Plan Do Check Act (PDCA) encourages bringing your staff into the process during the planning phase to brainstorm ideas. If they feel part of the improvement effort, usually the service improves. Measures actually help that happen. You can show your staff the numbers and graph the improvements. Most people react positively to the objectivity of measures.

Information allows you to assess where you are, where you want to be, how you will get there, and whether you have arrived. If, after introducing certain improvements, all the patients get their food trays in a timely manner, you know that your changes have been worthwhile and productive. Measurable goals show respect for the business, and measuring your goals shows respect for your staff. By measuring your goals you can monitor improvement objectively, improve the financial picture of your organization, and increase employee and customer satisfaction.

MANAGING WITH MEASURES

Let's move from food services to the population of pneumonia patients at a hospital. To improve care for these patients, what kinds of indicators should be developed? You would want to identify who the patients are (in terms, for example, of their age, geography, and comorbid conditions), the typical length of stay (LOS) for those patients, and the typical treatment. You might also want to know about complications and outcomes. As you begin to develop indicators, you are gathering data for a baseline that describes the present situation. The next step is to form a team, that is, a task force of stakeholders, and develop measures for improvements and changed processes.

The measures respond to your interests and questions. If you want to know how many pneumonia patients over seventy years old have the comorbid condition of heart failure or diabetes in addition to the pneumonia, you develop a measure that can answer that question. The numerator would be precisely the population you want to study, pneumonia patients over seventy years old who have the comorbid condition of heart failure or diabetes, and the denominator would be all pneumonia patients over seventy. Just as with the food services, once you understand the delivery of the service and identify any issues with providing excellent care, then you can tailor your improvement efforts to address the problem, and use measures to track the success of those efforts.

Defining a good hospital or a good process or a good physician also involves numbers and for similar reasons. Everyone can understand objective rankings. With resources so scarce and perhaps various interest groups saying their need is greater than others' needs, how does senior leadership know where and how to spend their limited money? Measures of care, processes, and outcomes can help administrators make these crucial decisions. But as I keep stressing, measuring without performing analysis or without taking action based on those measures keeps data removed from the process of improvement. Data should always be used to ask and answer pertinent questions related to improving care. Numbers help administrators and other leaders concretize their goals. For example, if mortality is above a specified level for a specific procedure, an investigation may be in order; pain should be below a certain threshold for treatment to be deemed effective. Thinking about a service or phenomenon in terms of numbers makes that phenomenon more manageable.

THE VALUE OF MEASURES

Establishing appropriate measures is becoming so fundamental to understanding the delivery of health care services that the CMS spends a great deal of time and resources carefully defining the numerators and denominators for evaluating the treatment of certain patients. The agency calls on experts from across the nation to serve on task forces that define the patient population so that every hospital will be able to measure the same phenomenon in the same way. The goal for the CMS is that health care providers will use the measures to improve care for certain patient populations. Because the CMS compares hospitals with hospitals and rewards hospitals that successfully treat patients according to its defined indicators, it needs to ensure that the measures are objective and clear.

The CMS has defined specific indicators for the care of such common conditions as AMI, heart failure, and pneumonia. Table 3.1 shows the quality indicators that caregivers for these conditions are asked to comply with and to document their compliance. According to the CMS, compliance with these indicators is equated with providing patients with quality care. Deviation from the indicators, then, defines a lower standard of care. Deviations include errors of omission, such as occur when a patient with an AMI is not given an aspirin upon arrival in the ED or a patient with pneumonia is not given smoking cessation counseling upon discharge.

The CMS is careful to specify criteria that define the appropriate patient population and that exclude patients who may not conform. Again, the goal is to compare treatment for the same patients across the country, to preclude the disclaimer that one organization's patients are sicker, have more comorbidities, or in any other way shouldn't be compared to others because they are somehow special. The same goal holds true when the state identifies risk-adjusted mortality rates for hospitals that perform certain procedures.

Once the denominator is carefully defined, that is, once the pneumonia patient is delineated, the numerator can track the intervention

Acute Myocardial Infarction	Jan	Feb	Mar	Apr	May	Jun	Jul	Aug	Sep	Oct	Nov	Dec
ACEI or ARB for LVSD												
Adult smoking cessation advice/counseling												
Aspirin at arrival												
Beta-blocker at arrival												
Beta-blocker prescribed at discharge												
PCI received within 120 min. of hospital arrival												
Thrombolytic agent received within 30 min. of hospital arrival												

Heart Failure	Jan	Feb	Mar	Apr	May	Jun	Jul	Aug	Sep	Oct	Nov	Dec
ACEI or ARB for LVSD												
Adult smoking cessation advice/counseling												
Discharge instructions												
LVF assessment												

Pneumonia	Jan	Feb	Mar	Apr	May	Jun	Jul	Aug	Sep	Oct	Nov	Dec
Adult smoking cessation advice/counseling												
Blood culture before first antibiotic												
Influenza vaccination												
Initial antibiotic received within 4 hours of hospital arrival												
Oxygenation assessment												
Pneumococcal vaccination												

Table 3.1. CMS Indicators for AMI, Heart Failure, and Pneumonia.

Note: ACEI: angiotensin-converting enzyme inhibitor; ARB: angiotensin receptor blocker; LVSD: left ventricular systolic dysfunction; PCI: percutaneous coronary intervention; LVF: left ventricular function.

or treatment. One of the CMS indicator measures for pneumonia patients is the administration of an antibiotic within four hours of arrival at the ED. Four hours is not an arbitrary number, but a goal based on EBM and developed through careful analysis of successful interventions for pneumonia patients. Those patients who received an antibiotic within four hours were healthier than those who didn't. In addition to promoting patient safety, the measure also forces physicians to behave in certain ways. To comply with the measure, they need to diagnose rapidly in the ED. Rapid and accurate diagnosis involves performing rapid triage and reducing patient flow problems, because rapid diagnosis moves the patient along the continuum of care rather than allowing the person to wait in the ED for a final diagnosis.

MEASURES AND ORGANIZATIONAL PROCESSES

Prior to the great push by CMS to establish treatment measures, there was little objectification and quantification of quality. The medical record, administrative data, and rules and regulations from agencies provided information, but there was no philosophical position that quality could and should be carefully defined through numbers and statistics. Therefore, what CMS was able to accomplish while helping to define the process of care for large populations of patients was to save lives—which was the agency's intent. If antibiotics were delivered appropriately and in a timely manner to pneumonia patients, the probability of survival was high. In addition, organizational processes were more efficient and improved because there could be no delay in triage and identification of disease, and so all the processes had to be timely and communication among the members of the caregiving team effective. With better processes and results, LOS is shorter, saving the hospital money and reducing the use of expensive, resource-intensive services (such as ICUs).

Interestingly, it is the CMS, an external agency, that is dictating to hospital administrators and physicians across the country how to deliver health care services. The agency has taken it upon itself to insist on efficiency and to force doctors to communicate across disciplines. Because it requires data, it is also enforcing the notions that care can and should be measured and evaluated and improved and that interventions and outcomes should be recorded as part of the medical record. Evidently, hospitals have not been able to move along these lines on their own. By developing standards of care, and enforcing measures, the federal government has changed the business of medicine in the United States. The initiative for medical management has moved from the individual physician and hospital to more objective and measurable standards.

Since the goal of the CMS measures, which are derived from the most up-to-date research, expert advice, and other components of evidence-based medicine, is to improve patient care and hospital organizational processes, you would think that everyone would jump on the bandwagon and be happy to comply with CMS recommendations for care and improvement. However, this is not the case. In fact there is a tremendous amount of resistance. Some administrators don't know about the regulations; some physicians don't want to be told what to do and resent being held accountable to an external agency. The physicians feel, and they may be right, that the government is trying to restrict their freedom. The medical record will clearly indicate to the government whether or not the hospital and the physician have provided the safest care. Yes or no. The audit is quite simple to do; the process is not.

CASE EXAMPLE: NUTRITION

Changing practices and internalizing new standards for care are difficult and time-consuming challenges. For example, most hospitals do not place much emphasis on ensuring that proper nutrition reaches the patient. Trays are dropped off; whether the food gets eaten or not, or even whether the patient can reach the tray, does not seem to be anyone's responsibility. Nutrition is vital to many patients—that they eat as well as what they eat and that they eat a special diet if they require it, as so many patients do. Yet somehow, perhaps because eating is such a normal, even mundane activity, it is not taken as a serious part of the health care experience and may not be perceived as part of the treatment plan.

But in fact there is an association between nutrition and decubiti, as well as other conditions. Yet it would be a remarkable organization that measures decubiti, notes a rise in incidence, and examines patient nutrition to see if there is a causal relationship. Again, perhaps because the measures for decubiti have become so routine, thinking stops at filling in a form for the measure. Nurses who are responsible for the documentation complain about the time spent on the paperwork when they could be giving bedside care. They write down the probability of decubiti for people at risk, and then . . . nothing. There is no follow-up. Their own documented evidence in the medical record remains unused and is not correlated to treatment.

The relationship between bringing a food tray and the patient's treatment is not typically perceived. But when a physician puts a patient on a feeding tube that is considered a serious medical intervention and appropriately monitored. When a patient is on a feeding tube, nutrition is suddenly hugely important to his or her well-being; prescriptions are written to supplement and promote proper nutrition, intake is noted and recorded, there are metrics associated with it.

If nutrition is important in one scenario, why would it not be important under more "normal" feeding conditions? Again, the answer is culture or a habit of mind. A feeding tube feels more like a medical intervention than delivering a tray. Patients generally get three meals and two snacks, adding up to five interventions daily. Yet no one watches to see if the patient eats because normal food intake is not considered medically interesting. But if a vitamin supplement has been ordered by the physician, the nurse waits to ensure that the patient in fact swallows the pill. Where is the sense in this distinction?

Basic needs, such as food intake, should indeed be considered important. In many hospitals food is perceived to be part of service quality, what is done to make the patient happy and comfortable, rather than a physical or medical issue. Often, however, because food is not considered important, patients go hungry. In my ED rounds I have seen patients waiting for twelve hours without food. Or patients are scheduled for procedures that require them to be fasting, and when the procedures are delayed, no one communicates to the kitchen that a late tray should be delivered or that the patient has not eaten. If that patient has a blood sugar or other condition affected by food, that lack of food could become a serious problem.

In response to patients' needs and concerns, today the government requires that nutritional assessments be included in the patient's history and physical and entered into the medical chart, especially to identify special needs. However, there is often a communication breakdown between the nurse who makes the assessment and the kitchen; because there is no systematic procedure, there is no follow-up. Developing measures could improve the process of monitoring nutrition. Expectations should be set and prioritized. Directors of various services should be brought together to brainstorm the relationship between food and other variables. Leadership should ascertain whether or not nutrition has an impact on LOS.

CASE EXAMPLE: HOUSEKEEPING

Measures are useful in promoting accountability for everyone involved in patient care and services. For example, a director of housekeeping wanted to know how her staff was performing—certainly a reasonable interest on the part of the manager. Because the health care system is heavily influenced by quality management methodologies, she was comfortable with the idea of developing measures related to her concerns. Knowing time is easily measured, and wanting information about the length of time it takes to clean a room, or to turn a room over, properly between patients, she began collecting data. How long *should* it take? How much time is *too* long?

> Control charts are quality control tools, initially developed by Walter Shewhart in the 1920s and popularized by W. Edwards Deming in the 1980s. Originally developed to monitor variation from industry standards, control charts can also be used to monitor variation from acceptable norms in health care. Once a norm is established, control charts can concurrently monitor whether there is excessive deviation from that norm or standard of care. By graphing variability from a predetermined standard, leaders can monitor when a process is *out of control* and take steps to address the problem.

After discussing issues of time with her staff, the director set expectations and established control charts showing upper and lower limits that the staff agreed were acceptable. Figure 3.3 illustrates a control chart for room preparation, with the upper acceptable limit at twenty-five minutes and the lower limit at fifteen minutes. The staff had determined that a room should be made ready within that time frame. Workers were tracked for four weeks, and their daily average charted. Figure 3.3 shows that at the beginning of the monitoring process Worker 1 and Worker 2 have a great deal of variation in the time they take to turn over a room and also from each other's time.

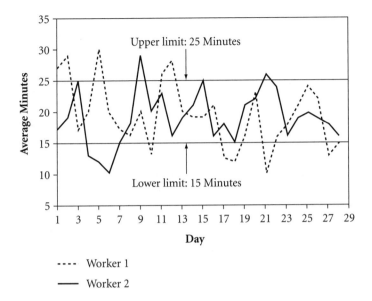

Figure 3.3. **Measuring Room Preparation Time Variation.**

By the end of the tracked period, their average is getting within the control limits and they also have less variation from each other.

This useful exercise in measuring average bed turnover time supplied the manager with information, information that replaced subjective impressions. She had a sense of what constituted efficient turnover and inefficient turnover, she was able to target further investigation to learn why there were certain roadblocks to a quick turnover, and she could focus efforts on improvement. She was able to quantify goals for her staff that were objective and comprehensible. The staff felt empowered because they had been involved in the process of determining the measure. The monthly report-outs detailed improvement efforts. Due to her leadership, the staff were clear about expectations and were not defensive about being held accountable for improved performance. As professionals, they too were interested in understanding what was interfering with maximum efficiency and in trying to improve.

The improvement process should not stop with one question, measure, or success. After gathering data on turnover time, understanding the roadblocks to success, and making improvements, the manager and the staff wanted to understand how the service they provided related to other aspects of the health care process. By collecting more data the staff realized that efficient bed turnover has an impact on waiting time in the ED, because if rooms were not ready, patients could not be released from the ED. Bed turnover time can also stall patients in the recovery rooms, because patients need to remain there until there is a room ready for them.

The staff realized that bottlenecks in the housekeeping process have serious clinical, organizational, and financial consequences. Patient satisfaction is also affected. There are also clinical consequences to keeping the rooms clean. When cleaning is inadequate, there may be an increased incidence of infection. When the rooms are not properly clean, patients may fall or have other incidents that could have been avoided. It quickly became apparent to the housekeeping staff how important their work was to the efficiency of the organization and how their piece of work related to the larger organizational goal—providing safe and effective patient care. Measures improved their understanding of their role in the delivery of care.

MONITORING PERFORMANCE

It is the role of leadership to set the tone for the organization. When leadership takes the CMS measures seriously, then the staff will also. Let's use one of the CMS indicators to illustrate how compliance improves patient safety and organizational efficiency. Assume that the leaders of an organization have made the determination to monitor aspirin administration, one of the CMS measures for appropriate care for patients with AMI. Evidence-based medicine has shown that aspirin reduces complications and even mortality for this patient population and that there is a relationship between timely aspirin administration and reduced mortality for AMI patients and between aspirin and more efficient patient flow (that is, leaving the ED).

However, the leaders discover that this seemingly manageable measure is being met with resistance. The physicians cite organizational obstacles, too much paper involved in documentation, and poor communication among different members of the staff. To provide the timely administration of aspirin involves accurate triage of the patient in the ED, and proper and immediate communication among the nurse, the ED physicians, and the patient's physician, who may not be able to get to the patient immediately to order the intervention and who may or may not agree with the ED physician on the diagnosis.

For the patient to receive good care, there has to be a close working relationship between the hospital-employed attending physicians (also known simply as *attendings*) and the community physicians, who may not share the hospital's goals or interests. Owing to the multiple caregivers involved, the patient doesn't "belong" to anyone. The nurse waits for the proper orders, the patient waits for admission to the appropriate level of care, the lab and radiology reports may refine the diagnosis, and the patient's private physician may need time to arrive at the ED to execute treatment. However, waiting delays giving the aspirin, and the four-hour marker may not be met.

This measure, like others, is not only about treatment but about timely treatment, proper diagnosis, and communication. The intent of the measure is to change clinical behavior and improve organizational processes. The measure is not an end in itself, to be used for reimbursement, but a means to improve the care of the patient and the organizational processes of the hospital by doing the right thing for the right reason at the right time.

MEASURES PROMOTE KNOWLEDGE

Measures can serve as a proxy for research. If you require information about clinical care or processes, you can gather it from objective measures. For example, if you want to determine whether or not it is effective and efficient to have a pharmacist in the ED to facilitate the delivery of appropriate and rapid medication to patients, such as aspirin for AMI patients and antibiotics for pneumonia patients, measures can help you determine the effectiveness of the pharmacist's presence. Data can be collected to determine whether the EDs with a pharmacist have patients with fewer complications and a shorter LOS or whether one class of patients benefits more from the pharmacist's presence than others. A measure provides an objective method of determining value added.

Among the reasons to acquire knowledge is to avoid problems. It is the responsibility of organizational leadership to identify and analyze problems, and not solely financial problems. Many administrators believe that if there are no serious adverse events, then there are no problems. Everything is running perfectly. But that's nonsense. There is always room for improvement in the delivery of care and its outcomes, and carefully defined measures can help hospitals identify and correct problems before they lead to terrible events or have to be reviewed by the quality committee or regulatory agencies. When patients or members of the board of trustees want data that show how a particular clinical process or intervention for a specialized population at the hospital compares to the national benchmark, it seems reasonable that the leadership should have these data. It would be unthinkable in the automobile industry, for example, to wait until a car was completely assembled before checking for defects and fixing identified problems.

The issue at hand is the recognition of the problem and the willingness of leadership to take responsibility for fixing it. For example, maintaining a clean environment has been proven, through clinical studies, research of the Centers for Disease Control and Prevention (CDC), and infection control practitioners, to be important for reducing mortality and complications. Yet during a financial crisis, among the first staff to be let go are the cleaners of the environment, who are (incorrectly) perceived to be unimportant to the hospital's operation. The second people to go are those who monitor and watch for problems and measure the level of cleanliness and performance based on evidence: infectious disease practitioners and quality management specialists.

LACK OF MEASURES LEADS TO POOR RESOURCE MANAGEMENT

The health care industry needs an overhaul of how business is done, and health care leaders need to commit themselves to providing a valued product to their customers. But many hospital organizations remain stuck in old and increasingly obsolete practices. For example, even a cursory examination of medical files reveals that the patient population is becoming more elderly, yet few if any organizational changes have been made as the demand for special services for the elderly changes.

It is easier to throw money at a problem than to carefully analyze its causes and develop changes. Often administrators do just that— buy new products in the hope of improving, but they do so without the information that would tell them whether or not the new product will help. For example, expensive specialty beds can be ordered for patients at high risk of decubiti, and these beds may indeed reduce the risk a bit. But if the measures continue to show a rise in the decubiti rate, then what do administrators often do? Buy more products.

Measures and databases can serve as proxies for intelligent planning and should provide an avenue for communication among different parts of the organization. When resources are spent without such information, there is a real risk that mistakes will be made. For example, let's say an elaborate expansion effort is underway at a hospital to provide outpatient services for a community, and facilities are bought and built according to information provided by the strategic planning division. Half a million dollars has been allocated for radiology equipment, space, and staff. However, quality management was not involved in the planning stages because project leaders did not recognize the value of collecting data in advance of delivering services. After the building program was begun, quality management staff asked planning leaders how many X-rays were typically done in a day, because the radiology suites were such a major expense.

No one knew the answer because no one had thought to ask the question! There was no information about radiology volume at all. After quality management collected data on outpatient services and radiology, it became apparent that allocating $70,000 would be more than sufficient to meet the needs of the community, yet over $3 million had been allocated. You wouldn't want to be the administrator who is forced to say a very red-faced "oops!" when that information goes before the board of trustees.

Looking at the entire picture helps hospitals avoid costly and poor decisions. Imagine that an outpatient mammography clinic has located a suspicious mass. For a biopsy to be taken, the radiologist has to mark the site of the mass, usually with special needles. The patient then goes to the surgeon for evaluation. What if these medical locations are not adjacent? What if no one thought this process through before the locations were established? Patients don't want to be traveling with needles in them, but this is exactly what happens unless someone has exercised some foresight. Yet many administrators avoid asking questions about clinical processes and collecting information about those processes until it is obvious that administrative mistakes have been made. Use measures to make changes. Otherwise it is very easy to make serious mistakes.

Here's another case in point. In an effort to reduce infection a hospital CEO made a decision to install new water filters. It would seem reasonable that prior to making that decision the hospital would acquire some evidence that connected the infection to water. It would be necessary to know, for example, what organism was responsible for some cluster of infections or whether many different organisms were involved. It would also be important to understand how the infection was transmitted, and if that process was affected by water filters. By collecting data, infection control monitors would be able to understand the present situation and create a baseline. When new technology (or a new service) is introduced, data can reveal whether the new equipment has any impact on reducing infection. Without either baseline or postintervention data, how could anyone evaluate the effectiveness of the intervention? Without adequate data collection and analysis, and in the face of a failure to reduce the infection rate, the administration might simply keep purchasing other equipment; this happens, but soon the organization's margin narrows.

When the delivery of services is efficient and effective, resources are being used appropriately. Measures help administrators determine efficiency. For example, if a problem intervention was to purchase new technology, measures would reflect whether the technology was effective in eliminating or reducing the problem. If the organization had been measuring various aspects of service before the problem, it has a baseline. Administrators can use the baseline to define future goals and determine the direction that the organization should move. However, technology is often purchased as a result of other considerations—persuasive advertisements or salespeople, the desires of special interest groups or high-volume physicians, or opportunities for reimbursement.

Different measures address different components of hospital organization: financial, operational, and clinical. Each component contributes to an understanding of quality, especially if traditional rigid demarcations are blurred. Measures help administrators understand issues of profit and loss in relation to issues of delivery of care and quality standards. For example, if an administrator wants to understand the financial requirements of, say, the cardiac services provided by the hospital, he or she needs information about the necessary equipment, current technology, appropriate LOS for specific procedures, patient case mix, complications, preventive measures against falls, infections, wound care, and the caregiving and support staffing required to support the specialized care necessary on the unit. That information can help a health care professional understand a clinical service.

MEASURES AND EVALUATING SERVICES

One of the mistakes administrators commonly make is to rely solely on financial data for information, whereas data about varied activities are interrelated, and so data in combination reflect more accurately the care delivery within the organization. A single measure, such as LOS, illustrates the complex relationship that exists among the variables. The CMS reimburses hospitals according to expected LOS for a specific diagnosis. For example, if a patient is admitted with pneumonia, he or she is expected to stay, and therefore the hospital will be paid for, a specific number of days. The hospital gets paid the same amount of money whether the patient stays less than or more than the expected number of days. Clearly, LOS is tied to revenue, which is why data regarding LOS are closely monitored.

Hospitals that discharge patients appropriately (that is, according to the standard schedule) or early are able to put another patient in the bed and receive income for that new patient. However, if a patient stays longer than the expected and reimbursed number of days, the hospital misses that revenue opportunity. Extended LOS costs the hospital money. It would seem obvious that it is advantageous—to the hospital organization, and the patient—to discharge patients early. However, if the quality of the care the patient receives is not balanced with the institution's financial expectations, everyone suffers. If a patient who is released early is readmitted with the same diagnosis, then there is no reimbursement for the second admittance. Or if a patient has to remain in the hospital due to infection or if a fall results in a fracture, then the hospital loses money. It is the hospital's responsibility to "do it right" (a JCAHO expression) the first time and to do it for the right reasons.

For an administrator, therefore, it is crucial to understand the clinical or operational reasons for a prolonged LOS or a readmittance, because both have a great financial impact on the organization. Monitoring quality measurements enables decision makers to understand and explain variations in LOS, to establish the relationship between what was expected and what actually occurred. If clusters of patients are staying longer than the expected LOS for certain diseases, it is important to analyze the situation and attempt to understand the reasons for it. Through measures, administrators acquire the ammunition to hold the appropriate people accountable. If the longer LOS (costing the hospital revenue) is the result of infection, quality measures can help the hospital identify the source of the infection, which in turn enables corrective actions to be taken to improve the situation.

Figure 3.4 represents the relationship between clinical care and LOS (cost). If there are no complications, a pneumonia patient should have a five-day hospital stay. On Day 3, if there are no obstacles to changing from intravenous (IV) to oral (PO) antibiotics, the discharge planning process should begin, and by Day 5 the patient should be discharged. A bell curve is used in Figure 3.4 to illustrate the financial cost of outliers, those patients who do not fall within the normal LOS range. Patients who stay only one day cost the hospital money because they underutilize expensive services and their short LOS suggests they had no need to be admitted and that they could have been given an antibiotic and sent home. Patients on the other end of the curve stay too long, and they also cost the hospital money because some complication occurred, such as an infection, and they cannot be released within the CMS parameters for reimbursement.

Focused analysis might reveal that infection is being spread due to poor sterilization techniques or even by some factor as mundane and uncomplicated as surgeons' not changing out of their street clothes before examining a patient. But until an administrator can link prolonged

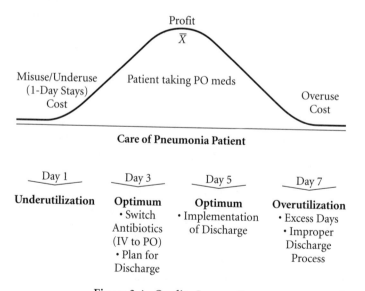

Figure 3.4. Quality Lowers Cost.

LOS, decreased revenue, infection, and sterilization practices, all these pieces of information will remain separate and uninterpretable. It is obvious that simply counting days and using a finance database would not help an administrator drill down to address the complex interrelationships among clinical quality, finance, and operations.

In order to understand the financial implications of treatment, an administrator needs to understand clinical processes, especially given that reimbursement is dependent on diagnoses and treatment (case mix index, or CMI). The more standardization in the delivery of care, the less variation from the expected course of treatment, the greater the revenue to the institution. The better the care provided to patients and the better the outcomes of services rendered, the greater the revenue returns for the institution. If, for example, patients from a certain nursing home arrive for hospital treatment with serious pressure injuries that will result in increased complications and a longer LOS, the hospital staff need to develop processes and procedures to address these patients' problems. But in order to address them, you have to know about them. Collecting information, in the form of measures and databases over time, will identify problems in care.

If processes in the operating room are efficient and if turnaround time is efficient, then the institution will reap more profits. If the care is superior and there are fewer complications, there is more profit to the institution. It is essential to understand where the profit lies in the process of care. A strong administrator understands enough so that he or she can plan intelligently for the future, can predict problems and proactively address them, and can balance resources required for different services.

SUMMARY

Health care institutions, like other complex business organizations, need to rely on data in order to

- Define value for their products.
- Improve market share by monitoring the provision of good services.
- Maintain the efficient use of resources.
- Ensure that patients receive evidence-based care.
- Reduce variation in treatment.

- Understand the relationship between interventions and outcomes.
- Measure abstract concepts, such as pain or a "good" hospital.
- Communicate leadership goals to staff.
- Compare one organization to similar ones across the country.
- Promote improved accountability from staff.
- Identify problems and evaluate solutions.
- Establish guidelines for the delivery of care.

Things to Think About

At the end-of-the-month budget meeting your CEO announces that the institution is not meeting its budget goals. Upon evaluation it is discovered that the number of orthopedic cases is decreasing and that in fact there has been a downward trend in new cases during the past year. The CEO is concerned and asks you, as an administrator, for your ideas to address this issue and to suggest improvements.

- How would you define the problem operationally?
- What tools would you use to evaluate the problem?
- What arguments would you bring to the CEO about the direction to take to improve the situation?
- What measures would you develop?
- How would you prioritize the multiple issues that contribute to this reduction in services?

CHAPTER FOUR

What to Measure—
and Why

I
n many organizations *quality* is a vague concept, and
one that is thought to be completely subjective and therefore unsci-
entific. However, quality can be objectified by developing clearly defined measures, collecting data about those measures, analyzing the
data, and communicating the resulting information to appropriate individuals. Quality measures, which are required by regulatory agencies, can offer health care leaders information to assess and improve
patient care and to ensure that they have timely, efficient, and effective care, with expected outcomes. Included in the definition of *quality care* is compliance with the CMS (Centers for Medicare and
Medicaid Services) evidence-based indicators (such as aspirin for
acute myocardial infarction, antibiotics for pneumonia, and smoking
cessation counseling at discharge). When measures are used quality
can be defined objectively and scientifically.

In this chapter I will outline how measures can be developed and
used to offer health care professionals, both clinicians and nonclinicians, information to improve the quality of care delivered in their institutions. I will also describe how the use of quality methodologies,
such as the PDCA for performance improvement, can provide a

framework for developing appropriate measures and for monitoring and improving various aspects of the delivery of care.

LEADERSHIP DETERMINES WHAT TO MEASURE

Leaders lead according to a value system, defining the kind of organization the institution should be. It is up to the senior leadership of the hospital to define the level of quality that is acceptable and the level that is not. Leadership defines priorities by answering such questions as these:

- What aspects of the organization are critical to its success?
- What expenses are most and least profitable?
- How can excellent patient outcomes be achieved efficiently and economically?
- What variables influence patient satisfaction?

These and many other factors need to be understood and balanced—through measures.

With objective criteria in hand, administrators have access to quality variables and can use factual information to make decisions. Becoming familiar with and using quality measures to deliver quality care helps the health care leader to do the right thing for the patient and to increase financial efficiency for the organization. The better the care, the fewer the complaints, complications, and incidents. When administrators understand how measures of quality reflect operational processes, clinical care, and patient services, as well as underlie good financial management, they become more comfortable about monitoring the delivery of care they are responsible for. Leadership and a strong quality management department should collaborate on using measures to understand the processes, procedures, and operations that have positive and negative impacts on patient care and organizational processes.

MEASURES DEFINE QUALITY CARE

Prevention is good medicine and helps the organization maintain its financial stability. Measures should be used to establish benchmarks for preventive processes—processes such as monitoring sterilization to prevent infection, providing fall prevention, preventing skin injuries, or reducing length of stay (LOS) through appropriate and timely antibiotic administration. For example, to decrease expenses, increase efficiency, and produce good to excellent outcomes, leadership needs to control nosocomial (hospital-acquired) infection.

Specifying the numerator and denominator of the measure ensures that it accurately reflects the information you want to collect. For instance, the general infection rate can be computed as the relationship between the number of patients who contract any infection within a month (the numerator, or N) divided by the number of patients admitted to the hospital per month (the denominator, or D). However, if the information you want is more specific, you define the measurement accordingly. If you are concerned about the incidence of sternal wound infections postsurgery, N becomes the number of postsurgical patients with wound infections over a specific period of time divided by the total number of surgical patients over that same time period (D). Once the measure is defined and the rate can be calculated, the information can be tracked over time. Collecting such measures allows an administrator to monitor trends, such as whether infection is rising, decreasing, spiking, or comparable to the national benchmark. Figure 4.1 illustrates the rate of surgical site infection in one hospital over a twenty-two-month period and shows that its rate is, by and large, lower than the national benchmark.

By carefully defining a measure, with the specific numerator for the objective of the study and the denominator delimiting the population of which the numerator is a subset, leaders can objectively and productively study performance, success, and opportunities for improvements. The data in Figure 4.1, for example, show that spikes in infection occur in the same months each year (January–February and September). With that information leadership can drill down in their data and attempt to analyze what might be contributing to the rise of infection during those months.

MEASURES INFORM
FINANCIAL DECISIONS

Data regarding the specifics of care help administrators make efficient financial decisions. For example, the nursing shortage in this country has resulted in staff vacancies that have had an impact on patient care. CEOs and senior administrative staff are expected to make hiring

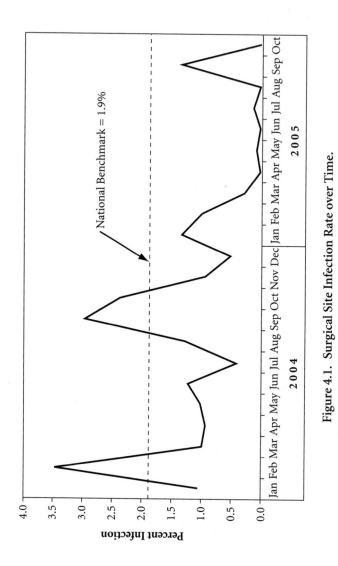

Figure 4.1. Surgical Site Infection Rate over Time.

decisions, but how? Using what information? In other words, what are the criteria for evaluating long-term versus short-term investment decisions? Hiring decisions obviously have an impact on the budget, but unless administrative leadership uses objective measures to look at the specifics of operations, evaluates the effectiveness of services, and gauges the effect of staff-patient ratios, how can they understand staffing requirements and the relationship between staffing and patient outcomes?

Many health care institutions are in financial difficulty because important decisions are being made without adequate understanding and information. Think of open-heart surgery and its huge requirements in terms of the operating room (OR), intensive care unit (ICU), specialized staff, and ancillary services and then compare those requirements to, for example, the treatment of patients with pneumonia, a far less resource-intensive hospitalization, assuming, that is, that the patient does not develop complications. Variables for both these conditions can be measured. Information (that is, data) about these variables gives administrators insights into the relationships among services, outcomes, and resource needs.

Tracking several potentially related variables can offer leadership important information. Figure 4.2 combines two variables, LOS and readmission within thirty days, across eight hospitals. If a patient requires readmittance within thirty days of discharge, it is possible that that patient was discharged prematurely or that the care was in some way deficient or inadequate. If administrators examine only LOS, they might believe that the shorter the LOS, the more efficient the hospital. However, if the hospital with a short LOS has a high rate of readmittance, as Hospital B does, then leaders may want to investigate and target improvements. Hospital D has both a long LOS and a high rate of admittance, suggesting inefficiencies of care that have financial consequences. Hospital G is providing the most efficient and effective care.

Because the government reimburses institutions according to the complexity of each case (using the case mix index, or CMI) and the procedures required to treat specific diseases, financial resources are dependent on clinical considerations and operational processes. For open-heart surgery cases, a measurable variable, such as turnaround time in the operating room, can have a financial impact for the institution. If the first procedure of the day is postponed due to operational issues, then for the rest of the day procedures are late. Late procedures have implications. It may become necessary to hire extra

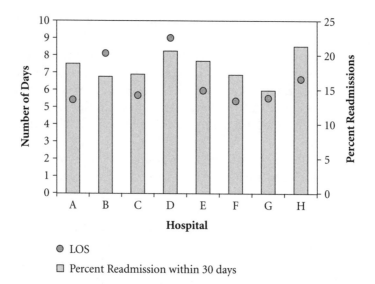

Figure 4.2. Length of Stay and Readmissions Within Thirty Days.

staff to work into an evening or night shift. Any complication during a procedure tends to cause expensive delays. Therefore good clinical supervision with clinical support can reduce such expenses. Ideally, a finance officer and a senior administrator learn enough about the delivery of care to ask intelligent questions and establish appropriate measures for data collection and analysis.

Tools and technology and even staff cannot be evaluated as a unidimensional financial expense. An administrator or financial officer can collect data in order to understand the complexity of services. For example, in the ICU there is usually a one-to-one patient-staff ratio. However, administrators may want to know if that ratio is crucial to the welfare of the patient, if the expense results in improved outcomes, or if it is simply a high degree of (perhaps unnecessary) monitoring. Analyzing measures helps an administrator discover the clinical as well as the financial value of a service. When leadership understands clinical care, financial decisions are not made in a void.

MEASURES AND PURCHASING DECISIONS

The financial implications of purchasing decisions are entwined with various aspects of patient care, and intelligent decisions cannot be made without an understanding of other expenditures and the impact on patient outcomes.

Administrators should consider using their quality management departments to mediate information between finance and the medical requirements of care. Quality indicators can help administrators determine the value of specific services, such as whether an elaborate (and expensive) CAT scan will result in better patient outcomes. Without data there is no way to assess whether more sophisticated technology should be purchased. With data, leadership can expect answers to such reasonable questions as what are the financial and clinical implications of a 64-slice CAT scan, and how will it be better for patient care than a 34-slice scan? The medical staff may request new equipment, but it is up to leadership to understand that equipment's relative value to the organization. Measures improve administrative understanding by providing detailed information.

Some decisions regarding expenses may have far-reaching implications, others may be of less consequence. Purchasing improved cardiac stents, for example, may reduce bleeding and complications from the stent procedure, so although this purchase is expensive it may result in fewer complications, a shorter LOS, and therefore a better financial situation than the hospital would have if the purchase were not made. Data collected over time would reveal the value, and leadership would be able to intelligently monitor costs and benefits. Likewise, robotics technology is very costly. Without objective data it would be difficult to determine if such an expense is of worth to the patients and to the hospital. Information can be collected about the volume of patients who might be attracted to the institution if robotic surgical procedures were in place and the outcomes were excellent. A financial assessment could be projected based on those numbers. Obviously, numbers provide a great deal of crucial information for decision making.

An example of a quality variable that reveals a great deal about operational and financial efficiency is mortality. Administrators should collect these measures monthly in order to monitor the delivery of care and the services being offered. If there are problems, for example, if there were three unexpected mortalities in the OR, there may be a problem that requires addressing. Mortalities cost money. Reports have to be filed with appropriate agencies; malpractice suits can occur; peer reviews have to be conducted. If the source of the mortality is infection, then corrective actions have to be put in place. If the source of the mortality is clinical incompetence, intervention or reeducation can be conducted.

But it is most important to know that the mistakes occurred and then to ascertain the causes in order to develop appropriate improvements. Administrators look at mortality reports and often go looking for someone to blame, rather than considering the situation as an opportunity to improve the delivery of care. If the hospital reports a high mortality rate for a specific procedure, such as cardiac bypass surgery, or for a particular patient population, such as heart failure patients, there might be a financial impact associated with that report because patients with these conditions or who need these procedures may be less attracted to the hospital. The public understands mortality data. (Physicians may say the data are flawed or not risk adjusted, but if the data are out there and the public is afraid, people won't come to the hospital for treatment.) Operationally, it may be important to understand why the rate is high so that specific processes can be targeted for improvement.

Quality issues and operational issues are interdependent. If data reveal that patients with certain conditions, such as elderly patients with AMI, have a higher incidence of mortality than others, then the care of that patient population has to be carefully reviewed. If patients from certain nursing homes die at a higher rate than others because those patients have comorbidities that are having an impact on mortality, then improving risk assessment might increase safety for those patients. These questions can be empirically tested through developing measures, collecting data, and analyzing trends.

MEASURES AND PATIENT SAFETY

Quality management data are required by agencies for accreditation and for compliance with regulations, but data are also collected as part of various national programs to assess and improve the quality of care, such as the CMS core measures, the Institute for Healthcare Improvement (IHI) 100,000 Lives Campaign, and the National Patient Safety Goals initiative of the Joint Commission on Accreditation of Healthcare Organizations (JCAHO) (see Figure 4.3). JCAHO mandates that each of its goals be implemented; the individual organization determines how to implement each goal. For example, to improve accuracy of patient identification, an organization is required to check two patient identifiers before administering medication, blood products, or performing clinical testing, treatments, or procedures. The hospital determines which two identifiers it will use. Improving communication involves ensuring that phone and verbal orders are properly understood; JCAHO recommends that hospitals require a *read-back* by the person receiving the order. Medication safety involves

2006 Hospital National Patient Safety Goals
1. Improve the accuracy of patient identification.
2. Improve the effectiveness of communication among caregivers.
3. Improve the safety of using medications.
4. Improve the safety of using infusion pumps.
. . .
7. Reduce the risk of health care-associated infections.
8. Accurately and completely reconcile medications across the continuum of care.
9. Reduce the risk of patient harm resulting from falls.

Figure 4.3. JCAHO's 2006 Hospital National Patient Safety Goals.
Note: Because JCAHO has retired some goals over the years as it has added new ones, the numbering of current goal sets is no longer consecutive.

several improvements: limit drug concentrations, review look-alike and sound-alike drugs to prevent interchanges, and label all medications. For infections, comply with CDC guidelines for hand hygiene. These goals and their implementation recommendations can be found at the JCAHO Web site (jcaho.org).

The data about safety are collected, and administrators should use the information to understand their operations; furthermore, because quality management data are benchmarked against national standards, administrative and other leaders can evaluate how their operations compare to other institutions. Through measures and benchmarks the data provide relevant information about daily performance and about areas where improvements should be instituted.

The IHI 100,000 Lives Campaign is the first national initiative to prevent avoidable deaths in hospitals and to implement change to improve patient care. The goal is to save 100,000 lives as of June 14, 2006. Highlights of the prevention program include the creation of rapid responses teams, using evidence-based care for AMI, preventing ventilator-acquired pneumonia, preventing indwelling venous catheter infections, preventing surgical site infections, and preventing severe drug events.

QUALITY METHODOLOGY FOR
PERFORMANCE IMPROVEMENT

Collecting data on an operational variable, such as blood administration, waiting time in the ED, turnaround time in the OR, or time to receive consultations or laboratory reports, reveals information about efficiency; efficiency has an impact on the financial success of the institution. In addition to using the quality management department to establish databases and benchmarks for best practices, the organization can use quality methodologies, such as PDCA and Six Sigma, that help analysts to inform administrators about services and to improve the delivery of care.

Using quality methodologies may enhance the assumption that excellent care is equal to a sound business plan and economic success. However, a simple economic model might even be in opposition to the mission of a hospital, which may be to serve the poor and the underserved. Such patients may not have the luxury of focusing on health prevention in the way that individuals with economic means and health insurance do. This lack of prevention might result in more sickness, which might in turn burden the hospital because it will be providing expensive care without reimbursement. Such expense can be anticipated, however. Therefore those expenses within the organization's control should be maximally efficient.

As long as the CEO is using a methodology that is based on data and statistical analysis, measures help employees and managers and administrators and members of the governance committees to share clearly defined goals that stem from a specific philosophical position and to share a commitment to excellence and improvement. Using any deliberate methodology creates a focus for addressing the process of care or product or service. With numbers, administrators can suggest, for example, improving the volume (that is, raising the numbers), eliminating wasteful services (as measured through volume and finance), improving productive services, and targeting specific goals.

Six Sigma is a methodological tool designed to reduce the negative economic impact of inefficient services. Based on the concept of the normal curve, Six Sigma was initially used as a measurement standard in product variation. In the 1920s, Walter Shewhart showed that three sigma from the mean is the point where a process requires correction. As a quality management tool for health care, Six Sigma is useful for analyzing and improving operational processes through measuring how far specific data vary from the mean.

For example, to understand turnaround time in the OR, data can be gathered about timeliness of patient preparation, OR readiness, equipment reliability, surgeon start time, readiness of appropriate ancillary staff, availability of required documentation, causes of delays, if any, and analysis of morbidity that might require extra OR time or an unanticipated return for repair. All of these variables can and should be measured, and each has a financial analogue. Once the inefficient process is identified, improvements can be developed.

The *Plan Do Check Act* (PDCA) cycle is a robust performance improvement methodology, and one that works particularly well in a health care setting. This model was also developed for monitoring quality improvement in industrial settings and is designed to standardize processes and minimize variation, that is, eliminate mistakes and rework. The PDCA cycle, by breaking function and role into variables that can be measured, helps leadership understand the clinical and medical environment and the method of providing care.

Using the PDCA cycle to continuously improve quality allows current performance to be measured, processes to be analyzed, and improvement actions to be identified (Plan). Improvement actions are then implemented (Do), and the benefits of the actions are measured (Check). Once measured, improvements can be standardized and communicated and reassessed (Act). The PDCA cycle provides for the systematic acquisition of knowledge through focused data collection and, through measurements, validates that improvements are effective (see Figure 4.4).

There are many advantages to using an industrial performance improvement model, such as PDCA, to continuously evaluate improvement and determine variation from the standard. The PDCA cycle provides a continuous loop of quality monitoring, based on data from measures. By defining the numerator and denominator of a measure, leadership can objectively understand the product being delivered, and by holding staff accountable to these measures, leadership clearly anticipates a uniform standard of excellence.

As with most complex activities, doing something according to a plan is more productive than simply reacting to some stimulus on the spur of the moment. In health care, planning involves collecting information and analyzing current processes, identifying gaps in care, establishing improvements, and monitoring their effectiveness. Making improvements or changing processes is often met with resistance and confusion over accountability (who is in charge) and details of the process changes (who is doing what).

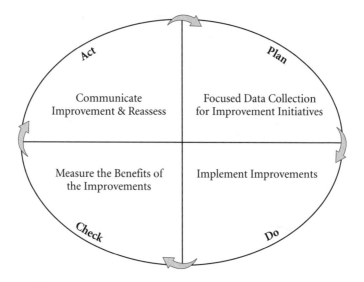

Figure 4.4. A Quality Improvement Methodology: PDCA.

My experience shows that to improve a process, adopt new information, and actually change the delivery of care, the unit manager and the clinicians benefit by working within a methodology, such as the PDCA, that continuously and objectively reviews and evaluates their actions. The PDCA method allows the professionals to pause and consider the workload with a critical eye. Working with many patients, with multiple diagnoses and treatment plans, caregivers require a method that directs and prioritizes activity. Daily planning must be continuously communicated, from the beginning to end of shift, through the changes in shift, and to the end of the shift to maximize efficiency and reduce potential for errors.

DEVELOPING A PERFORMANCE IMPROVEMENT PLAN

Every aspect of the PDCA cycle depends on measurements, not of an individual's experience but of a population of patients. The first stage, Plan, requires that stakeholders, who have similar goals, formulate an assumption about care, in other words, develop a hypothesis. The hypothesis may be derived from external or internal sources. For example, because the CMS requires smoking cessation counseling for pneumonia patients, administrators may assume that most of the patients are receiving the recommended counseling. Their assumption may be that clinicians are incorporating patient education about smoking into their practice.

Data can be collected to confirm that assumption. Quality management can develop a methodology for chart review and determine the percentages of patients who have had the counseling and of those who haven't. With this information in hand, further analysis can drill down in the data and examine the records of those patients who did not receive counseling to see if they have any areas in common, such as physician, unit, secondary diagnoses, and so forth. However, without quantifying the process, it is hard to convince anyone that there is a problem, let alone that it should be fixed.

The assumption or hypothesis should reflect areas of concern to the investigating team. Another assumption might be that patients who are given antibiotics before surgery have fewer infections than patients who are not given this medication. This is a testable assumption. Other testable assumptions are that patients who develop pneumonia on ventilators were not properly weaned off the ventilators, and that patients who fall do so because of a desire to be mobile when there are insufficient staff to assist them. Administrators and staff should meet together to determine which assumption to measure and which care process to improve.

In the planning stage organizational culture should be evaluated to determine whether there are possibilities for change and whether a structure exists to implement changed practices. Leadership chooses which battles deserve to be fought; not every process needs to be changed, and different stakeholders may be interested in different issues. Physicians may be concerned with high mortality, surgeons with infections, nurses with falls, and respiratory therapists with ventilator-associated pneumonias. It is up to the administrative leadership to determine priorities, perhaps based on the goals, mission, and vision of the institution or derived from external pressures from the public and the media or revealed on some scalar dimension by such questions as which problem poses the highest risk, where can the impact of improvement efforts be greatest, or where can financial gains be seen? The senior staff of the organization decides priorities for improvement, what outcomes to look at, what processes to change, which measures to use, and what process to develop to monitor, assess, analyze, and communicate the results of the data collection activities.

Before you determine your measures it is essential to define your clinical or operational goals, establish priorities, and understand the patients (the organization's customers) and their concerns and priorities. The quality management department at our health system developed a prioritization matrix to help decision makers evaluate competing issues for performance improvement (see Table 4.1). Competing issues for improvement are listed across the top of the matrix. Each issue is evaluated by the criteria listed along the side of the matrix—such as alignment with leadership goals and vision, impact on the delivery of care, or outcomes showing a negative trend. Different organizations will define their criteria differently, but it is useful to think about prioritization in terms of structure, process, and outcome. For each issue a value is entered in each cell of the matrix, from 0 to 3 (no application to maximum concern) and these values are totaled. A comparison of the totals defines the most pressing priorities. By ob-

	Evaluative Criteria	Issue 1	Issue 2	Issue 3	Issue 4	Issue 5
Structure	Governance/board of trustees (is it aligned with the vision?)					
	Finance (that is, cost/budget)					
	Meeting benchmarks (CMS, IHI, JCAHO, DOH)					
Process	Operation (how we treat patients/delivery of care)					
	Evidence-based medicine					
	Is the issue (associated concerns) measurable?					
Outcome	Trending in negative pattern					
	Compliance (is it a deviation from practice?)					
	Patient satisfaction surveys/patient complaints					
	HMOs/denials					
	Malpractice rates/insurance premiums					
	NYS DOH incidents					
	Issue total					

Scale: 0 = no application; 1 = low concern; 2 = moderate concern; 3 = maximum concern

Table 4.1. Prioritization Matrix.

jectifying and quantifying priority options, stakeholders have an opportunity to evaluate and consider how to allocate resources.

In the Plan stage the stakeholders should be able to realize that change is possible and that change would be good for the institution, the patients, and themselves. Even this initial point may be difficult because often caregivers see no need for improvement, an attitude that there is no reason to fix what isn't broken. Tradition—doing things the way they have always been done—makes people comfortable. However, acquiring data usually reveals that improvements should be made.

When the senior staff agree on priorities, develop assumptions about performance improvement, and assign responsibilities for roles and functions within the organization, the Do phase of the cycle begins. The stakeholders of a process or procedure determine the improvement. For example, surgeons may want a better assessment for administering antibiotics in a timely way. When weaning protocols are being reviewed, the pulmonary physicians and the respiratory therapists are the stakeholders, as well as the nursing staff. If falls are being investigated, perhaps a multidisciplinary committee can develop an improved risk assessment screen for patients who are at high risk for falls. The Do phase is where a change is designed and relevant measures (numerators and denominators) are defined to monitor the process of change and the improvements. Also in this phase, procedural details are developed, such as which staff members will be collecting data for the measure, how the data will be collected (in what form) and reported (to whom), who will analyze the data, over what period of time, and how the results of the analysis will be reported out and to whom.

As always, the measure is defined by what the stakeholders want to know. If mortality rates are at issue, then the group may want to look at various procedures and have analysts analyze mortality according to various clinical services, patient populations, treatment, and diagnoses, whatever is of interest to leadership and staff. It is a good idea to review the literature for existing methods of data collection and analyses. Established studies can become benchmarks for the standard of care.

Once the design of the measure and the data collection efforts have been accomplished, improvements and changed practices are designed and implemented. The Check phase of the PDCA cycle is used to monitor the new procedures and to see if they are successful. New measures may need to be developed, such as the timing of antibiotic administration. During the Check phase it is important to keep monitoring the improvements to ensure that they are maintained. This phase is the evaluation phase, in which the program under study is assessed. It is useful to ask the stakeholders and the medical board for input, in order to increase confidence in the improvement efforts.

In the Act phase, changes are implemented, a procedure that requires administrative commitment. During this phase a table of measures can be developed that will provide a snapshot of improvements (or the lack thereof) over time. In this stage it is also important to effectively communicate information about changed processes throughout the organization, from the bedside workers to the members of the highest governance committees.

CASE EXAMPLE: PLAN DO CHECK ACT FOR BARIATRIC SURGERY

In the health care system where I work, because we have a strong quality management department with databases that promote measures and that are respected by physicians and administrative leadership, quality management was able to conduct an improvement initiative related to bariatric surgery, that is, surgery for the treatment of obesity. Improvement was driven in this case from within the organization.

The more an experience can be quantified, the better it can be understood. Quantifying experience also promotes accountability of staff because expectations are clear, standards are defined, variation is discouraged, and most important, it is obvious that someone cares and is monitoring what is happening. When a multidisciplinary system task force determined that various aspects of bariatric surgery needed to be carefully evaluated, the task force realized that there would be an advantage to using a deliberative process, such as the PDCA cycle for performance improvement.

In the Plan phase the objective was to protect the safety of this patient population, which is highly complex physically, socially, and psychologically, and to develop guidelines. This relatively new surgery has risks that can result in complications, a dysfunctional life, and even death. Specific standards of care had to be explicitly defined for this procedure. For example, although many general surgeons wanted to perform the procedure in their hospitals, as it is an innovative and high-demand surgery and has the potential to be lucrative for the physician and for the hospital, not all surgeons were qualified to perform bariatric surgery. Therefore guidelines for physician credentialing needed to be developed. Moreover, the results of surgery were not only related to the technical ability of the physician but to the patient's ability to comply with dietary protocols for weight management. Therefore communication among the nutritionist, social worker, psychologist, and surgical team was as important for a successful outcome as the procedure itself.

In the Do phase, assessment and credentialing issues were addressed. A multidisciplinary task force was convened and charged with developing a method to implement a safe and low-risk environment for the patient, determining the specific requirements for credentialing physicians, and establishing a consistent methodology for appropriate patient identification, selection, and assessment. The task force was composed of specialists from quality management; physicians, including bariatric surgeons; community physicians; the chief medical officer; the chief of surgery; pulmonologists, for input into sleep apnea; anesthesiologists, for input into airway management; radiologists, regarding the limitations of and alternatives to diagnostic testing equipment for this patient population; intensivists; nurses; nutritionists; psychologists; psychiatrists; and social workers. The health care team ensuring patient safety wanted patients and families to recognize that this procedure alters a patient not only biologically but also through its powerful impact on psyche and lifestyle as well.

For over two years the team researched the available clinical literature, brainstormed many issues, and came to consensus on specifications of appropriate and safe care. This effort resulted in the development of guidelines for volume-based credentialing of physicians, for assessment for appropriate patient selection, and for patient counseling, institutional requirements, and staff education. Because the guidelines were based on evidence-based practice, care was standardized and measurable, from the presurgical physician's office visit to one year postoperatively. A specific algorithm for clinicians was developed, the bariatric surgery clinical pathway, which could be used to standardize care (see Figure 4.5). This *CareMap* documents, on a single page for each day, whether or not specific consultations, tests, treatments, medications, and much more have been met or remain unmet.

Once guidelines were established, the Check phase was begun. The quality management department, in collaboration with the multidisciplinary task force, created a database to monitor relevant indicators from presurgery to one-year postsurgery for ongoing review. The

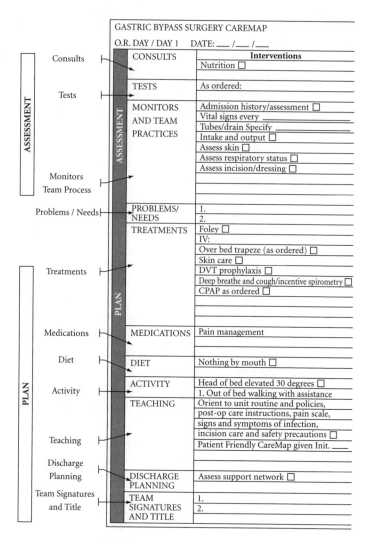

Figure 4.5. Bariatric CareMap.

outcome database, approved by the system hospitals' medical boards, is used to evaluate each program through the use of common data definitions and uniform numerators and denominators; it tracks and trends patient demographics, outcomes, and complications (see Table 4.2 for one example of an outcome database).

Objective outcome measures analyze patient outcomes. The guidelines seek to prevent serious postoperative complications (such as deep

Outcomes

Patient's abnormal lab values are addressed.
Met: ☐   Unmet: ☐   Initials:
Patient's abdominal dressing is dry and intact.
Met: ☐   Unmet: ☐   Initials:
Patient is hemodynamically stable.
Met: ☐   Unmet: ☐   Initials:
Patient's urine output is above 300cc every eight hours.
Met: ☐   Unmet: ☐   Initials:

3.	5.
4.	6.

Patient understands the need for DVT prophylaxis.
Met: ☐   Unmet: ☐   Initials:
Patient demonstrates correct use of trapeze.
Met: ☐   Unmet: ☐   Initials:
Patient's skin integrity is maintained.
Met: ☐   Unmet: ☐   Initials:

Patient's pain is adequately managed.
Met: ☐   Unmet: ☐   Initials:

2. Patient tolerates increased activity, out of bed walking with assistance.
Met: ☐   Unmet: ☐   Initials:
Patient/significant other verbalizes an understanding of the plan of care, unit routine and policies.
Met: ☐   Unmet: ☐   Initials:
Patient verbalizes an understanding of the post-op course and treatment.
Met: ☐   Unmet: ☐   Initials:
Patient verbalizes an understanding of the pain scale.
Met: ☐   Unmet: ☐   Initials:

3.	5.
4.	6.

Figure 4.5. Bariatric CareMap, Cont'd.

vein thromboses). A standardized program was created through consensus; lessons learned and best practices were shared and then implemented across the health care system. By reviewing the data and employing objective standardized definitions that were compared to internal and external benchmarks, accountability was increased, as was communication among the board of trustees, the hospital medical boards, and the physicians. Improved communication also served as a

Indicators	2003	2004	2005
Pre-op nutrition assessment completed (%)			
Post-op psychiatric assessment completed (%)			
Post-op wound infection (%)			
SICU/SCU LOS			
Hospital LOS			
Return to OR within 30 days, excluding infection			
Post-op blood products			
Return to OR for bleeding			
Mortality			

Table 4.2. Sample Bariatric Table of Measures.
Note: SICU: surgical intensive care unit; SCU: special care unit.

tool for teaching about the risk and benefits of the procedure. The process spurred the medical boards to develop specific standards of care around the procedure, especially around different weight categories.

The Act phase includes ongoing education for the relevant specialists across the system. The Center for Weight Management, under the psychiatry department, provides comprehensive weight management services for patients and their families and offers educational programs to staff. Psychological and sensitivity training and education are also made available to ensure competency among nonphysicians. The latter program is directed specifically toward this special patient population and its physiological as well as psychosocial risks. Teleconferences have been held that addressed sleep-disordered breathing and obesity and also morbidity and mortality.

The result of this initiative was improved patient care and more efficient organizational processes that resulted in decreased cost to the hospitals and the system. Because complications went down, the LOS for patients was shorter. The readmission and reoperation rates were low. Patients were appropriately screened, assessed, and educated and received follow-up counseling and support. Staff were objectively credentialed, and education was provided for staff in various specialties—nursing, surgery, anesthesia, nutrition, and psychology. Staff were encouraged to share their experiences and lessons learned in an open and blame-free environment, and this facilitated discussion about such controversial issues as the particular requirements for adolescent surgery and surgery on the super morbidly obese (patients weighing over 500 pounds).

The bariatric surgery initiative also informed capital investment decisions to upgrade facilities and to acquire appropriate equipment according to a principled and deliberate set of criteria. As each hospital created a bariatric center, new physical environments were established with special operating rooms, beds, and wheelchairs. Patient support groups were created and the transfer of information from the physician's office to the hospital is now seamless. Goals were developed for each institution to obtain JCAHO Disease Specific Certification or designation for having standards of excellence as endorsed by the American Society of Bariatric Surgery Centers of Excellence Program, a designation that attracts patients. Some hospitals sought both.

MONITORING VARIATION FROM THE STANDARD

The PDCA cycle for performance improvement was originally designed to minimize defects in production. The theory is that if products are made according to a standard, every product will be perfect. Lack of perfection is equivalent to variation from the standard. In health care, also, variation from the standard serves as a red flag that there may be a defect in the process, that is, a defect in the delivery of an intervention or an unanticipated outcome. As in industry, the goal of performance improvement is to minimize defects in processes. Delivering safe and effective care is good business. Trying to react to problems after they occur or to correct bad practices that have become entrenched costs more money than adhering to standard (evidence-based) guidelines.

Through the use of measures processes can be explained. The population is clearly defined, as is the service under evaluation. The measure is a proxy for the specific service performed, with the numerator defining what is being done and the denominator defining the group that the service is being performed on.

Organizations can also ensure compliance with standards by spending money on consultants. But if regulations and evidence-based indicators are understood for what they are—standards of excellence—everyone involved can be encouraged to internalize each standard and to do it right, before expensive events or complications occur. Measures create efficiencies and better care outcomes. By measuring variation, leadership develops criteria with which to objectify the distance between the gold standard of care (defined by evidence-based medicine) and actual practice. The wider the gap between the two, the poorer the care, and the more expensive it is to provide this substandard care.

Let's define the health care product as removing an infected appendix before it bursts. If you remove it in a timely way, that's the standard of care; if you do not, there could be serious complications. The standard of care is also to avoid removing a healthy appendix. With measures, it can be determined how many false positives occurred in the hospital, how many erupted appendixes happened, and why and with what outcomes. Before determining how best to approach patients with appendicitis, it is important to evaluate the current practice. A measure can be developed and tracked over time. Once you have a sense of the scope of the problem, and the volume of patients involved, a multidisciplinary group might study the literature on appropriate standards of care for appendicitis. Research is valuable because relying on the experience of one or two physicians may be inadequate. Their experience may involve too few patients to make accurate generalizations. If data from evidence-based medicine are used, you have the advantage of learning from large numbers of patients, from many physicians, and from many reports of the best treatments and the adverse events that may occur.

If data reveal that indeed there have been instances of erupted appendixes in your organization, it may be useful to develop an algorithm of care with the goal of avoiding this terrible situation. The algorithm would detail criteria for identifying the problem, and outline the appropriate actions to take. Consensus can be established on whether to use physical impressions, such as abdominal pain, lab results, such as elevated white count, or radiological results, such as CAT scans, to determine the diagnosis. Health care experts may decide that the algorithm should include three indicators for a diagnosis of appendicitis and that if the patient has two then the surgeon might consider the evidence and act quickly. The algorithm would then be monitored to see if it is successful, and if so, it becomes the standard of care throughout the organization. Such work can be based on even one occurrence of a burst appendix.

Even one adverse event costs a hospital large amounts of money in follow-up care for complications, malpractice claims, and poor public relations. By internalizing the idea of providing patients with value, everyone benefits. When an adverse event occurs, it is important to do a root cause analysis to determine the gaps in care and the risk points. You can be sure that if a problem occurs once, unless it is fully understood, it will happen again. You don't want to be in the position of having to face the patients, families, and media and explain why there are problems that endanger patients in your hospital. You want to always anticipate potential problems, using measures to monitor care. With measures, as soon as you see a blip in the data—a rise in infection, for example—you can send in a SWAT team of analysts to figure out what is going wrong and develop corrective actions. Senior leadership should not only commit to measuring variations in care but also build the PDCA, a planned and deliberate approach to continuous quality improvement, into the culture. When leaders expect forethought, the staff will deliver.

CASE EXAMPLE: MOVING BETWEEN LEVELS OF CARE

Maintaining standards and monitoring variation promotes improved organizational processes as well as better clinical care. The following example illustrates how recognizing defects in care and establishing improvements benefits the patient and the organization.

Management of LOS for elderly medical patients can be predicted to some extent based on past experience (that is, data) with this population. Their needs in terms of mobility, posthospitalization care, and physical and psychosocial issues can and should be planned for. However, care of the elderly is usually not planned for well. Often their needs, other than for medical intervention, are not identified upon admission. This is unfortunate because any issue or problem may increase over time, especially if it interacts with medical problems.

One of our community hospitals receives a large number of admissions from a particular nursing home. Several years ago the hospital received a letter of complaint from that nursing home saying that when its residents had to be hospitalized, they were returning to the home in worse shape than they were when they left. Leadership responded to this issue by replying that indeed, over time, the elderly patient does get worse, regardless of medical intervention. In other words, the care the hospital was delivering was appropriate and the patient population was at risk. However, when a second complaint was made, warning that the nursing home would refer patients to another institution, the CEO asked the quality management department to look into the matter more scientifically.

Data revealed that the nursing home complaint was valid, that patients were indeed returning to the nursing home with less mobility, with decubiti, with infections, and with depression—objectification of the notion of "worse." Although the hospital physicians had adequately dealt with the specific medical problem that brought each elderly patient into the hospital—for example, the patient who arrived with a fever or a high white blood count did receive antibiotics on time—there was little, if any, attention to any other factor. The patient's physical condition deteriorated because there was no communication between the nursing home and the hospital about the multiple needs of the patient.

Further quality management research found that the physical environment of the hospital was not particularly suitable for the elderly patient, and therefore patients were at increased risk for falls. The food was not appealing and was perhaps left out of reach, and therefore patients were not eating. With their nutrition suffering, patients were not properly absorbing their medication. Care providers were not monitoring that the patients were mobile enough to ward off skin injuries, and therefore patients suffered from decubiti and complications of decubiti.

Once these specific issues were identified, changes were made in the process of care. Clinical staff received education about caring for the elderly patient, specifically improving environmental factors, risk assessment for falls and decubiti, and nutritional counseling. In addition to these improvements communication between the nursing home and the hospital was improved. Information was transferred about the physical and psychosocial needs of the patient as well as the medical problem that required hospitalization.

The transition between the nursing home and the hospital became smooth, and the patients returned to the nursing home with appropriate and improved health status. It was the CEO who, responding to the nursing home complaint, led the charge to change the process, to identify the problem, and to correct it. The physicians and the nursing staff changed their clinical outlook to improve the delivery of care. The intervention of the CEO was focused on the process and the operation of providing care among institutions, that is, patient flow from one level of care to another.

UNDERSTANDING PATIENT FLOW

Patient flow has a financial impact on the hospital, and patient flow can be deconstructed into individual and measurable parts that can be monitored for improvement. It is obvious that the more efficiently patients are moved through their episode of hospitalization, the greater will be the advantage to the hospital and the higher will be patient satisfaction. Leadership needs to supervise patient flow, and the most productive way to do that is via measures. Figure 4.6 outlines the levels of care in a typical episode of hospitalization. When administrators understand patient flow and can identify bottlenecks in the process, they can then collect information about the impact on services, on the budget, and on clinical outcomes. Once problems are identified, relevant improvements can be implemented.

Generally, patients enter the hospital through the ED. Hospitals don't get paid for extended ED stays, yet many EDs function almost like a hospital unit, because, for a host of reasons, it is difficult to move patients from the ED onto one of the hospital's regular units. Measures can be collected that reveal waiting time in the ED, the number of potential patients who left without being evaluated, and the time from triage to diagnosis to admittance to a unit. If these data reveal that the time is prolonged, other data can be collected about the cause of the delay. Are delays caused by waiting for consults, for lab work, or for reports or by other technical issues, or are they due to housekeeping or transport bottlenecks? If the ED is overcrowded and patient care is delayed, what contributes to the congestion and impedes efficiency? Without measures, one might conclude that the ED is short-staffed, but there are many other possibilities. Table 4.3 shows a table of measures with examples of ED variables that could be collected and reported to senior leadership to assess the delivery of service. If the ED is crowded and patients have to wait for a long time or are otherwise dissatisfied with their care, they may not return. By tracking information over time, leadership can locate where the delivery of care has fallen short of the standard. It's a buyer's market, and so if leadership wants to attract patients, care has to be competent.

If housekeeping is not able to make up a clean room so that a patient can be moved from the ED onto the unit in a timely way,

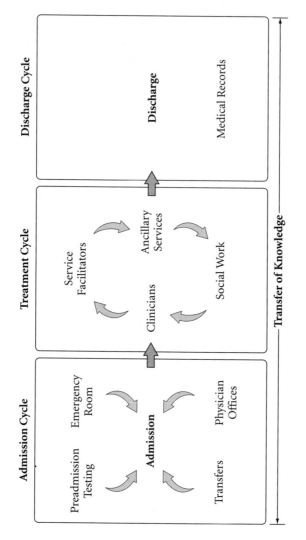

Figure 4.6. Patient Flow.

Indicators	2003	2004	Rating
Left against medical advice rate	1.47	1.85	*
Left without being evaluated rate	2.37	2.39	**
Returns within 72 hrs. and admitted rate	45.27	28.67	***
Mortality rate	1.2	0.6	***
Mortality within 24 hrs. rate	0.5	0.2	***

Ratings

*** Performed better than the previous year

** No change from previous year

* Performed worse than the previous year

Table 4.3. Sample Emergency Department Table of Measures.

improvements can be made. Once the problem is identified, a new process can be developed to improve turnaround time, resulting in better care for the patients, greater efficiency for the ED, and financial improvement as patients move appropriately to different levels of care. Data can be collected on how long it takes for laboratory test results to be received and how long patients remain in the ED awaiting those results.

With everyone working independently to meet the goals of his or her own department or service, regardless of the other departments or services, interdepartmental communication may be weak. Each department's objective might be met, but not the whole organization's. To change this, staff in departments involved in any way with ED patients must work with consciousness of their impact on patient flow, rather than focusing solely on their own department's goal.

There may be many reasons that patients remain in the ED longer than clinically appropriate. Measures can help administrators pinpoint where processes should be improved. For example, if the discharge planning process is not begun appropriately, it may be another source of extended stays. Data on processes will inform administrators about bottlenecks. All these measures of care are also measures of effectiveness, efficiency, and thus financial viability.

It is important for administrators to supervise the throughput process and not let segments of the process act independently of each other. This means that administrators are not focused just on the ED but on radiology, housekeeping, dietary, and so forth, as well. All services have to understand their role in patient flow. The movement of patients along the continuum of care within the hospital must be analyzed daily in order to locate points that force the patient to stay in one place longer than necessary.

Quality and operational measures lead to financial success. When the care is smooth and timely, then the laboratories; technical processes; ancillary services; and environmental, housekeeping, and nutritional services—as well as clinical services—are all working effectively and efficiently. In addition, the communication structure of the performance improvement committees, if used appropriately, reinforces this success.

SUMMARY

Measures and databases

- Reflect leadership priorities.
- Respond to external and internal requirements.
- Reflect best practices.
- Are founded on evidence-based research.
- Should be realistically accessible for collection and analysis, with explicit numerators and denominators.

The quality management department should help administrators develop databases and consistent measures and help leaders determine best practices in care. When the leadership supports the data collection and analysis efforts, clinical staff will follow suit. Valid measures help to standardize assessment across various units of the hospital or across institutions in the health care system. Everyone agrees on the same numerator and denominator. Apples are always being measured against apples, and not against anything else.

It is important to involve the relevant stakeholders in the definition, collection, and analysis of the measures and to use a deliberate methodology, such as the PDCA, for performance improvement. Consistent measures can be replicated over and over again—in different environments and for varied periods of time. Measures have to be reasonable and collectible and about something someone cares about.

Things to Think About

There is a sudden spike in infection among surgical patients. The local newspaper is warning people to stay away from the hospital where you are a top administrator. How would you manage this issue?

- What measures would you develop to identify the source of the infection?
- How would you interpret the results of the data about the source of the infection, and according to what standard?
- What process would you use to develop an improvement plan?
- Which stakeholders would you involve in the process?
- What data would you collect to monitor the improvements?
- How would you communicate with the media about the improvements?

CHAPTER FIVE

Promoting Accountability Through Measurements

I n a health care institution, as in any business, people have to be responsible for their own activities and for the activities of those they manage. In a hospital accountability moves from the bedside caregiver up the ranks to the board of trustees. The board is, in turn, responsible to the community that the institution serves (see Figure 5.1 for an example from a hospital system).

Board members are entrusted with organizational oversight, a responsibility that has traditionally translated into maintaining the financial viability of the organization. If the organization is in the black and making a profit, then the hospital and its leadership are successful. If it is not, then they are not.

However, financial measures do not always capture important information about the delivery of care or provide meaningful explanations of errors and events. Moreover, financial measures do not insulate leadership from criticism. If the media report a devastating medical error or a higher-than-expected mortality rate, and the community is understandably upset, the board may conclude that leadership is not doing its job well. Good outcomes, as defined by such measures as a low infection rate or low mortality rate, may require

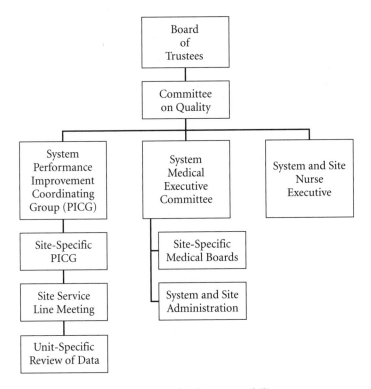

Figure 5.1. Levels of Accountability.

substantial financial investments. Therefore an administrator should be able to justify such expenditure as essential for good outcomes.

In this chapter I will discuss how information can be used to understand gaps in the delivery of care and how preventive oversight can prevent harm. By monitoring and analyzing adverse events and communicating information about specific problems in the delivery of care throughout the organization, health care organizations can improve patient safety and organizational efficiency.

MEASURES AND ORGANIZATIONAL GOALS

Measures can be gauges not only of clinical processes but also of values; they are a way to examine the process of care, to look at methods and outcomes, and to learn from errors and events. Information and education help the decision maker relate practices to goals and understand guidelines for care. If, for example, self-extubations result in infection, and if infection results in a prolonged length of stay (LOS), patient care is not optimal and the hospital loses money. Poor care and cost go hand in hand. If there is a wrong-site surgery, patient care is substandard, and if the event results in a major malpractice claim, the hospital loses money. Leadership defines what is of value and what standard to set for the delivery of care. When adverse events are reported, leaders may believe it is easier for them to say that care is complex and tragedies happen than to insist that every patient should have the safest possible outcome. However, it is safety that usually results in financial benefits for the organization.

Measures assist health care leaders in monitoring their goals. If it is your goal to increase patient satisfaction, you need some way to assess that satisfaction—that is, some measure. You might create a scale for satisfaction and collect information from patients and then aggregate the responses in order to know the satisfaction level in general. If you had a 95 percent rate of patient satisfaction, you might want to know why the other 5 percent is not meeting the standard. To investigate this, you need more information—that is, more measures. You can drill down and collect information about the particulars involved in the notion of *satisfaction*. Because you don't necessarily have that information, you can ask the staff—the front-line workers, the people who interact with patients directly—if they can help you establish measures. They might say food, cheerfulness of staff, quiet at night, and so on. You can collect information on the 5 percent and determine if there is a common indicator of dissatisfaction. Unless you gather information, and analyze it, you have no way to understand the reasons for satisfaction, the levels of satisfaction, and the reasons for dissatisfaction.

This example reveals certain important issues about measures. Someone has to ask questions or have goals, those goals or questions have to be reasonably measurable, those measures have to be reasonably collectable, and the resulting data have to be analyzed for a purpose—improvement.

JUSTIFYING EXPENSES

If the CEO or senior leadership say they will tolerate nothing more than a 0 percent infection rate in the hospital, that number has to be understood as an objective, a value that can be translated into a willingness to put resources into infection control and prevention, no matter how low the rate is. If there are frequent malpractice claims against the hospital or if the state department of health is called in to review adverse events, the board of trustees may require an accounting from senior leadership. Therefore it is important for leadership to have the tools to explain to the board and others about the delivery of care so that they can offer an intelligent and appropriate response to the concerns.

Quality data are useful tools because they can translate care into objective and comprehensible terms. If the hospital CEO reports to the board that the self-extubation rate in the institution is below the national average, how would a board member know how to interpret that information? It is not necessary to go to medical school to realize that if a patient is not properly weaned from a ventilator and inappropriately pulls out the breathing tube (that is, self-extubates), adverse complications can ensue. There could be pain, infection, or pneumonia.

I know a CEO who became interested in the specifics of self-extubation when his mother went into a nursing home and was put on a ventilator. Due to his personal interest, the CEO made it his business to ask questions about ventilators, and because he had answers to those questions, he was later able to explain to the board the importance of establishing weaning protocols for safe and timely extubation, of collecting data on self-extubation and associated complications, of analyzing indicators related to ventilator use, such as the types of procedures and patients that require ventilators, and of understanding the complex issues involved in self-extubation.

Such a level of understanding is a far cry from simply reporting that the self-extubation rate in the hospital is 2 percent, a number that doesn't reveal much information. Saying the rate is below the national average does not communicate a great deal about patient safety either. Even if physicians find fault with the measures, claiming that differences in percentages are not significant, an administrator, and certainly anyone who has a loved one on a ventilator, can argue that no one should pull out his or her ventilator tube inappropriately or prematurely if programs and processes can be devised to prevent that from happening. With data in hand, leadership can articulate why a weaning protocol is being developed by a multidisciplinary team of stakeholders, why such a protocol is important, how the operational processes of the hospital would be affected, and how patient safety would be improved. In general, information helps to explain that money is being well spent.

CASE EXAMPLE: SELF-EXTUBATIONS

When the leadership of our health system expressed concern about intensive care unit (ICU) expenditure and asked quality management to assess whether utilization of this expensive hospital resource was appropriate, a performance improvement initiative was begun, using the Plan Do Check Act (PDCA) methodology, and involving the major stakeholders in the project. A systemwide committee was formed to evaluate critical care services, with a membership of quality management leaders, intensivists, ICU directors, ICU nurse managers, and respiratory therapy leadership from the ICUs at several of the system hospitals.

The committee adopted specific goals for improvement:

- Standardize critical care quality indicators for monthly collection and analysis.
- Develop admission and discharge criteria for the ICU.
- Improve and monitor nursing competency.
- Formalize protocols, such as for weaning from ventilators.

After meeting and researching ICU care for a year, the committee found that there was indeed inappropriate utilization of the ICU, with many patients using ICU beds without needing ICU services. The committee further concluded that leadership was lacking, competency required improvement, and policies needed to be defined, standardized, and formalized.

Among the first priorities for the committee was defining indicators for data collection, in order to establish consistent measurements to develop a critical care database. A uniform set of measures would track and trend data for important areas of care over time, such as admission information, acuity of illness, LOS, ventilator use, mortality, and unplanned (that is, self) extubations.

Figure 5.2 details ICU mortality rates for sepsis patients over a two-year period. Based on the APACHE (Acute Physiology, Age and Chronic Health Evaluation) III score, the data compare the actual mortality rate with the predicted rate at comparable institutions and also against a national database for this patient population.

Each hospital collected data on these specific indicators. Individual hospitals used these data to identify where they required improvement

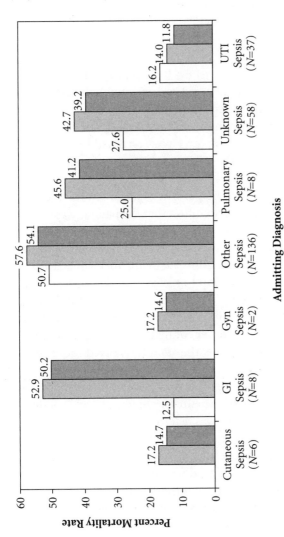

Figure 5.2. ICU Mortality Rate for Sepsis Patients, 2004–2005.

Note: GI: gastrointestinal; Gyn: gynecological; UTI: urinary tract infection.

efforts and where the care was successful. Analysis of data revealed a great deal of variation in self-extubation rates across the system ICUs, ranging from 3 percent at one hospital to a high of 17 percent at another. Because there are serious complications associated with mechanical ventilation, it is important that clinicians detect the earliest point that a patient can breathe without the assistance of a ventilator. Patients can self-extubate for several reasons. They can be ready to breathe on their own, which suggests a failure by staff to extubate the patient in a timely fashion. Another explanation for self-extubation is that patients may be inadequately sedated and thus agitated.

Self-extubations were tracked through the critical care database at each hospital, and each incident of self-extubation was evaluated to discover the cause. A special task force was convened to improve the care of ventilated patients in the ICU, and this group developed a special review tool for analysis of self-extubation events.

Data analysis revealed that 66 percent of the unplanned extubations resulted from a lack of recognition that the patient was ready to be weaned from the ventilator. This information provoked the task force to develop sedation and weaning protocols, which were standardized across the system after approval by the medical boards.

Data helped hospital leadership to realize the advantages of using the protocol and encouraged ICU leadership to adopt it. The data demonstrated that those hospitals that used the protocol had fewer self-extubations and therefore fewer complication and infections; they released patients from the ICU earlier and thus saved more money than those hospitals that did not use the new protocols.

Staff education, including grand rounds for physicians and in-service education for nurses and respiratory therapists, was conducted for the new weaning protocol. It was determined that respiratory therapists could be appropriately trained to implement the weaning protocol and thereby facilitate timely extubations, which then resulted in a reduction of self-extubations. This decision had an impact on staffing of ICUs. The adoption and success of the weaning protocols led to a steady decrease in unplanned extubations, and the rate has remained below the national benchmark over the past eight years (see Figure 5.3).

This improvement project required that changes be made in multiple units at multiple hospitals with different leadership and serving different patient populations. Using data to build trust and consensus was most effective. Leadership support for the improvement initiative was also crucial for ensuring its success. Defining, collecting, trend-

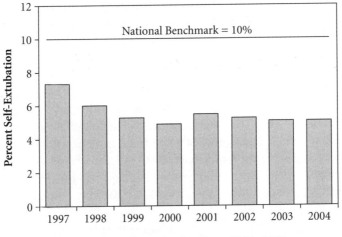

Figure 5.3. Self-Extubation Rate, 2004–2005.

ing, and communicating quality data replaced subjective and variable care practices with objective standards for optimal care. Through clearly articulated policies and protocols that facilitated more rapid weaning of patients from ventilators, the self-extubation rate was reduced and patient safety improved.

Accountability for maintaining the standard of care is reinforced though the quality management databases. Critical care data are distributed and reviewed through the performance improvement group for the system. Comparative analysis among the hospitals quickly identifies best practices and opportunities for improvement. Through the use of standardized protocols and uniform measurements for care in the ICU environment, utilization of resources has been significantly improved.

GETTING THE DOCTORS ON BOARD

With measures, administrative leadership can hold the clinical staff accountable for care along objectively measurable dimensions, and especially for compliance with recognized evidence-based indicators. Even if you are doctor to the stars, if you score low on mortality rankings or other measures of poor outcomes, that has an impact on your reputation. If physician data show higher than expected mortality, it is important for leadership and for the physician to ask data-driven questions: Who are the patients (demographics)? What comorbidities are associated with those who die versus those who survive? What was the process of care? Were there issues of competency? Were decisions made that were not in keeping with protecting the patient's safety? Data stimulate investigation and provide opportunities for physicians to reflect on their practices.

Physicians have to be intellectually open to accepting a change in culture, moving from a culture that values individual and individually interpreted success to one that values compliance with evidence-based medical practices. If pneumonia patients are not given antibiotics, for example, and evidence shows that elderly patients who enter the emergency department (ED) with pneumonia go quickly downhill without an antibiotic, the physician has to answer for the noncompliance that is documented on the medical record.

Leadership has the challenge of holding the physician accountable. Private attendings, particularly in small community hospitals, to avoid coming to the ED out of hours, often rely on secondary sources for diagnosis rather than primary ones (that is, themselves). What typically occurs is that physicians ask the ED staff to "rule out" a diagnosis (such as pneumonia) by using tests and technology, before the physicians come to the ED at their routine time and make a diagnosis themselves. When an aspirin is indicated, the physician might prescribe it over the phone. However, in the case of an antibiotic, appropriate for pneumonia, the physician might wait until the next day when he or she arrives for rounds. According to the guidelines of the Centers for Medicare and Medicaid Services (CMS), the next day is too late to administer an antibiotic to maintain maximum patient safety.

Moreover, what may seem a straightforward practice—give pneumonia patients an antibiotic within four hours of arrival at the ED—may be difficult to implement for operational reasons. In order to comply with the timely administration of an antibiotic, the physician has to be present to make the diagnosis, the tests have to be done quickly, the results have to be communicated promptly, and a pharmacist has to be available to service the ED at all times. If the patient is diagnosed quickly and treated appropriately and in a timely way, then the patient can leave the ED for a hospital unit, a process that involves other types of organizational oversight to manage such issues as bed turnover, housekeeping, and patient throughput.

For the administrator the timely delivery of the antibiotic is not only a patient care issue but also an operational and financial issue, because data reveal that delaying antibiotic administration for patients who need it causes a prolonged LOS and results in use of extensive resources. The cost of care becomes higher than the reimbursement payments. In general a "rule out" diagnosis means that the patient remains in the ED without care delivery.

Some physicians rebel against standardized indicators, complaining that evidence-based medicine compromises their autonomy and requires cookie-cutter treatments. It is my belief that those physicians are unfamiliar with the relevant literature and are allowing their egos to trump their intellects. However, a majority of physicians are becoming educated about measures. They want to provide quality care; that's the service they are selling. Data should be used to focus on care decisions. For example, the CMS expects antibiotics to be administered to all pneumonia patients within four hours. This is a measurable phenomenon: either the antibiotic is documented as given or it is not. Expectations are clear. And institutions must document compliance with this recommendation in order to get paid.

These kinds of recommendations specifically detail how to protect patients. Because the recommendations are coming from the outside, external to the physician and the hospital, they are forcing a cultural change. Physicians are being held accountable to national standards of patient safety, and data are collected about the success of meeting those standards.

Physicians should abide by evidence-based recommendations, not because this is required but because it has been proven the right thing to do. Administrators should apply pressure on reluctant and noncompliant physicians to change their practice because it is required, because it is the right thing to do for the patient, and because the hospital is rewarded financially when they do. Using measures of compliance with evidence-based indicators helps to change attitudes. Success can be measured on both an individual and institutional level. When the data show that compliance with indicators is low, then the organization gets a wake-up call. At some point an administrator has to say, this is not OK. Then change comes. The pressure of measures is that they provide a yardstick for the evaluation of care, objectively.

CASE EXAMPLE: WRONG-SITE SURGERY

In addition to assessing care through measures that detail the delivery of care, health care organizations can be alerted to inefficiencies and to dangerous practices through analysis of adverse events or incidents. The following example illustrates how event analysis can be used to provoke changed practices.

Wrong-site surgery is an avoidable tragic event that has attracted national attention. External agencies, such as the Joint Commission on Accreditation of Healthcare Organizations (JCAHO), the National Patient Safety Initiative, the American College of Surgeons (ACS), the New York State Department of Health (NYS DOH), and the Agency for Healthcare Research and Quality (AHRQ), among others, have attempted to eliminate wrong-site surgery by recommending processes, procedures, and guidelines that should be followed to avoid this error. All of these organizations, and my own experiences, stress that primary among the causes of this error is the failure of the surgeon and the surgical team to communicate with each other, as well as their failure to follow the guidelines established by the hospital to ensure patient safety. The reasons for these failures are difficult to identify. The cultural assumption that the surgeon is infallible and cannot be questioned still exists in many operating rooms; the surgeon's belief that his or her training supercedes recommended guidelines for conducting the surgery is also at fault.

Let me recount a hypothetical case that is based on authentic events, although I am disguising some of the facts for reasons of confidentiality. An elderly man had a mass diagnosed on the left side of his brain and was scheduled for a biopsy. The hospital policy in place to ensure correct site surgery includes the consent to surgery, which details the operative site; confirmation by the nurse with the patient about side or site; verification of the operating room (OR) schedule that includes site or side; site or side verification documented correctly on the patient's plan of care; and initials of the surgeon, nurse, and anesthesiologist confirming the procedure and site. Wouldn't these multiple verifications and confirmations seem to provide safeguards for the patient?

However, an error was made. During the surgery for the preceding case, the nurse questioned the surgeon about the upcoming procedure, and the surgeon verbally indicated the side—incorrectly. It was to be the last case of the day, and perhaps he was hurried or distracted. Responding to the surgeon's words, the technician prepared the OR, positioning the instrument table for a right (incorrect) side biopsy. The preanesthesia assessment, which requires site verification, was not conducted. The right side was marked in the OR with a line, and the patient was prepped (shaved and positioned) for the incorrect procedure.

Everyone involved reacted to the (incorrect) position of the table and preparation of the patient. No one verified the site, either through documentation or radiological sources, as the protocol demanded. Furthermore, proper procedures require that before the surgery, there should be a pause, and surgeon, anesthesiologist, and nurse are expected to explicitly articulate which side is supposed to be worked on. Use of a pause as a safety measure is recommended by JCAHO to improve patient safety and promote accountability of the professional staff, because they are expected to verbally specify the correct site. When this case was investigated, it was found that although required, this pause did not occur. No one involved questioned the surgeon, although subsequent analysis revealed that the circulating nurse and the resident were aware of what the correct side was. However, they assumed that the surgeon knew better. The surgeon performed a biopsy of the right side of the brain, and not until he was writing up his notes of the operative procedure did he realize his error!

Had the surgeon followed the prescribed policy for site verification, this error would not have occurred. Had the other professionals questioned the surgeon, this error would not have occurred. The surgeon believed that the policies in place somehow didn't apply to him. Although he knew that he had to sign a form, which is supposed to be signed after checking various documents in the OR, he signed it beforehand. Clearly, it was a meaningless piece of paper to him and not a method of ensuring safety for the patient. It is devastating for a physician to discover this kind of terrible and avoidable error.

This case shows that it is not sufficient to develop policies and procedures unless there is physician commitment to follow them, what is called *buy-in*. External agencies can require various safeguards—multiple signatures or pauses or cross-checks of various sorts—and yet, unless these requirements are taken seriously and responsibly, they are just another annoyance to be undermined or ignored. The entrenched culture of the OR is very difficult to change, and administrative and clinical leadership are challenged to pressure physicians to follow the spirit of the requirements, because doing so preserves patient safety. Professional arrogance and a hierarchical culture get in the way of change and of safety.

Shockingly, this case is not especially unusual. JCAHO, which keeps track of serious incidents, has analyzed many wrong-site cases and has identified various risk factors, among them multiple surgeons, multiple procedures, unusual time pressure due to organizational rather than clinical issues, and unusual patient characteristics, such as obesity, that might require unusual equipment or positioning.

Reviews of wrong-site surgery cases revealed that failures of communication were the primary cause of these events, especially a failure to confirm with the patient during the consent process or during the physical marking of the site, and incomplete or inaccurate communication among members of the surgical team. Analysis of cases also revealed failure to review the medical records or imaging studies. Flaws identified in verification procedures were the absence of oral communication in the OR, the unavailability of relevant information, the exclusion of some members of the surgical team from the verification process, and the attitude that the surgeon should never be questioned. JCAHO stresses the value of using multiple fail-safe procedures, such as marking the operative site after confirming it with the (preanesthetized) patient and requiring every member of the team to confirm the site and, by initialing the record, to be accountable for site accuracy.

JCAHO is not the only organization to alert organizations to the risks of not following procedures. The NYS DOH has also published detailed guidelines that stress the importance of communication among the surgical team members. The ACS has published guidelines for physicians to use to implement controls to eliminate this problem, and AHRQ has published a patient fact sheet so that patients can protect themselves from wrong-site surgery. Once again, patient safety is the focus of attention due to governmental intervention rather than internal self-monitoring of hospital physicians. The public will not tolerate wrong-site surgery, and accordingly, governmental agencies are pressuring hospitals and health care organizations to monitor, measure, and report such errors.

Poor performance in the OR on site identification may be the result of physicians expressing their independence from administration. By insisting on accountability from physicians, the administrative and governing bodies can help to change the culture.

ANALYZING ERRORS

One of the reasons to continuously measure various aspects of care is that monitoring data can alert leadership when processes begin to fail. When mistakes occur a root cause analysis is required by the state. Root cause analysis is a quality management tool designed to help people understand and reduce defects and maintain a safe environment. Through a careful analysis of an event, the variables that led to the event can be identified, and then processes can be put in place to improve. During a root cause analysis the major categories of causes that may have contributed to the event are identified. Usually these categories include environmental factors, human resources, policies and procedures, technology, and so forth. Once the major categories are identified, the analysis can become more specific.

A cause and effect diagram, sometimes called a fishbone diagram or an Ishikawa diagram (after its inventor, Kaoru Ishikawa), is a tool that illustrates graphically how various factors have an impact on a particular result, or outcome. Complex problems, such as wrong-site surgery, usually have several primary causes, which can serve as categories for detailing the smaller issues. Using a cause and effect diagram, analysts can categorize the large "bones" of the diagram and reveal what factors contributed to the adverse outcome.

The more detailed the analysis, the better. Data can target where a mistake was made. Most root cause analyses reveal that it is rarely one big error or a single incompetent staff member that results in an adverse event. Usually, there is a kind of domino effect, where one small mistake leads to another small mistake until eventually there is a big error that could have been prevented at several spots in the overall care process. Those vulnerable spots need to be identified, but this is difficult because they do not always seem serious in and of themselves. Measures should be developed to monitor whether surgical safety improvements, such as the pause, are actually implemented and performed consistently over time.

In addition to proving to the state and JCAHO through a root cause analysis that the organization understands how an error occurred, it is also mandated that the hospital present a corrective action, that is, a plan that will avert the problem. The quality management department can assist department leaders in the root cause analysis and formulating appropriate corrective action plans. Regulatory agencies check whether an error was an isolated incident or the result of faulty systems, such as an unsafe environment or a lack of competency or education. They review how the problem or event was handled: what changes were introduced, who approved the changes, and whether the medical board and the board of trustees understand what happened. Everyone involved in caring for the patient has to be accountable for safe care.

Administration, responsible for the safekeeping of the patients and the smooth running of the hospital, has to understand and support the improvement efforts. An error means that something broke down in hospital operations, and when that breakdown becomes public, as it invariably does, it is very bad public relations. Further, there can be malpractice suits, and then insurance rates increase.

CHANGING THE CULTURE

An organization's measures reflect the goals and the philosophy of its leaders and often the goals and philosophy of the officials who represent the public. Issues surrounding the reporting of data about medication errors provide an example of how a focus driven by external sources can lead to a change in hospital culture.

There are two commonly accepted definitions for a measure of medication error, a major safety issue. Medication errors can be measured against the number of prescriptions given each month or against the number of patients in the hospital. If you use the former measure, you will look great. The rate of medication error will be low, minuscule, because the denominator will be huge. But don't pat yourself on the back yet; the problem is that the measure is not revealing what you want it to, whether improvement is needed to reduce errors. If the goal of your measurement is to assess problems and make improvements, then you use the measure that actually reveals errors. The second measure will have a smaller denominator and be a more valid indicator of problems. The definition of a measure depends on the leadership's goals, values, and philosophy.

The medication delivery process has many potential opportunities for errors to occur. The physician has to correctly diagnose the problem and accurately and legibly write a prescription. That prescription then has to be accurately transcribed and correctly communicated to pharmacy. The pharmacist has to correctly fill the prescription. Then the correct medication has to be brought to the correct unit, and it must be correctly labeled for the correct individual. The nurse then has to correctly administer the medication to the correct patient. Typically, pharmacists monitor medication errors, but only those errors that they are in a position to catch, such as prescriptions that have been transcribed incorrectly or potential interactions with other medications or allergy alerts. The pharmacist has little control over the process once the medication leaves the pharmacy. Therefore, as the measure is developed, extensive education should be implemented to show that medication errors are the result of a complex process and a system with multiple potential defects.

Any variation from the norm, from guidelines that define the standard of care, can be defined as an *error*. When there is an adverse incident, such as occurs when a patient is given the wrong dose of medication, there is a report, and it is obvious that there was a problem that requires correction. But what about the patient who does not receive an aspirin on time—is that a medication error? In our system the medical board is starting to consider it as such and to ask for an action plan. Omission is an error too, especially when the evidence illustrates that giving an aspirin to an acute myocardial infarction patient can save his or her life.

It is vital that errors be monitored and measured. However, few professionals want to admit to incompetence or even inattention, and so potential errors and near misses are frequently underreported. If quality management collects the data and analyzes it, the process may be more objective because this department's goal is to understand the complex process of medication administration and to improve it. By breaking down the analysis, quality management can classify an error by type of severity, class of drugs involved, and the location in the hospital where the error occurred, and can identify where in the process of delivering medication problems exist.

Medication error was exposed as a huge problem by the Institute of Medicine and other organizations, yet hospitals were not reporting a high rate of error. To improve this situation the New York State Commissioner of Health put pressure on hospitals, in the form of fines, to report their medication error rate more accurately. The result of her attempt to get organizations to identify and report their errors was successful, and the rate of errors reported was greatly increased. By addressing underreporting head on, the commissioner challenged the culture of silence that surrounds poor outcomes and poor processes. It is certainly understandable that organizations are not eager to expose their problems to public scrutiny, but unless problems are quickly identified and directly addressed, they don't get better and can even get worse. The commissioner used the measure of medication error rate to force institutions to improve care by identifying and tracking medication problems as well as by developing corrective actions.

By forcing accountability for errors through objective measures, the commissioner helped to change hospital culture. When leadership uses the measures, they are taking the position that examining the process of care is important and that identifying problems and making corrections must be part of the culture. It was the commissioner's point of view that in order to provide a safe environment, administrators needed to know about and face up to the problems that they had in their organizations. An effective and objective tool for doing this consists of measures and benchmarks; the benchmarks express the goals of the organization—where it wants to be and what level it will be satisfied with. Benchmarks can be flexible. It might be an idealistic benchmark to have zero medication errors, but nonetheless that benchmark sends a powerful message to the caregiving staff.

Administrators can be held responsible for errors because it is their job to design and provide a safe environment; to run the organization efficiently (which means without errors); to provide patients with good outcomes, because that is the service they are hoping to purchase; and to maintain a positive financial balance. A medication error affects the organization and is a blemish on the institution, reflecting badly on administrative capability to control the process of care and its environment.

The nursing staff can also be deemed responsible, not only for errors but for underreporting potential errors. When medication is about to be administered incorrectly by one nurse and another notices and prevents it, the damage is controlled and perhaps the offending nurse is taught to be more careful. Rarely is a formal report filed, as it is supposed to be. However, when units do not report these near misses, or close calls, a climate is created that incubates a larger problem, one that could result in serious patient harm. When, instead, organizations fix small problems before they become bigger ones, everyone benefits. If the error or near miss is reported in the formal way, then the information can be shared and new processes instituted.

It is precisely this knowledge that a series of seemingly trivial gaps in care can easily lead to adverse events that has encouraged hospitals to report near misses, those errors that never reached the patient but if they had would have resulted in a problem. Reporting near misses also raises the consciousness of caregivers about dangerous practices.

Figure 5.4 graphs the medication error rate and the report of near misses over a one-year period. In January, the medication error rate is high and the reports of near misses low. However, after a year promoting the importance of monitoring and reporting near misses, the near-miss rate has increased and the medication error rate has decreased, due to conscious monitoring of preventable errors.

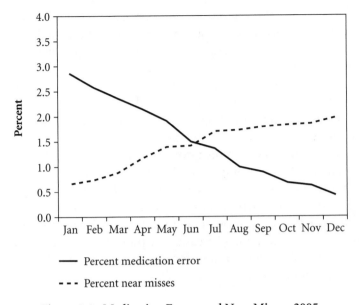

Figure 5.4. Medication Errors and Near Misses, 2005.

ASKING QUESTIONS

Accountability can come from asking questions that require answers that are quantified. For example, if you are the administrator of a behavioral health unit that employs psychiatrists and is a so-called closed unit, and there has been a serious incident, let's say, an elopement that resulted in harm to the patient or others, it is your responsibility as an administrator to ask questions—and to expect your staff to have answers. You might most reasonably ask, is elopement a common problem on this unit? To answer that question, numbers, that is, quantifications, are required: how many patients does the unit serve, and of that number, how many elopements have there been, over some specified period of time?

Wanting further detail, you might ask whether elopements are associated with some particular treatment, diagnosis, or physician. To answer that question, comparative data are required. You might also want to know the procedure that is presently in place to prevent elopements, and what is causing that procedure to be ineffective. To analyze the process, you may need to collect more data. Finally, you may need to know what the appropriate response is to an elopement; what steps are taken? As an administrator you don't want the public or the media asking you these questions if you don't have any staff that can provide you with answers.

Ideally, leadership shouldn't wait for an incident to analyze the delivery of safe care. Data should be obtained and measurements devised proactively. Having data readily available enables an administrator to ascertain whether a particular elopement was a unique or rare phenomenon; if not, the administrator would certainly want to question the staff about why a common problem has gone unresolved. Unless administrators ask questions, answers will not be forthcoming. Measures provide concurrent watchfulness and review of care, retrospective analysis and problem identification, and also proactive and prospective identification of areas where problems can develop. Competent leadership does not wait for a crisis to begin to ask questions and gather information.

EVALUATING INFORMATION AND COMMUNICATING RESULTS

Once an improvement effort or changed process is identified, it is important to develop accurate and reliable measures to monitor the effectiveness of the improvements over time. Communication is critical if change is to happen. Performance improvement committees are useful for identifying gaps in the delivery of care from different perspectives, and can serve as internal consultants for reviewing processes of care with a critical eye. Using an existing committee structure for this purpose has the further advantage of maintaining established lines of communication throughout the organization. Every month, in our health system, during performance improvement meetings, measures are presented and improvements evaluated.

Regulatory agencies hold physicians accountable for the delivery of care by monitoring and requiring medical record completion, because the medical record is the best source of evidence about how the patient was managed during an episode of hospitalization. Further, by examining medical records in the aggregate, agencies can gather information on operational efficiency. Although clearly important, completing the medical record does not seem to be critical to many in leadership positions; they are satisfied as long as the rate of completion is above

JCAHO's requirement. Without a leadership commitment to this task, physicians can think themselves too busy to fully document their delivery of care. However, the medical record is the primary source of data for how the organization is managed and documentary proof that patients are safe.

SUMMARY

Questions involve measures. Goals involve measures. Success is defined through measures. Failures are counted with measures. Improvements are recognized through measures. Databases bind all these issues together. The organization can determine to adopt certain measures and administrators can determine to hold staff accountable, but for the measures to have the desired impact (that is, improved care), the senior leadership has to promote their value to the institution. When the CEO expects that compliance with measures will be 100 percent, it makes a difference. However, the CEO simply does not have authority over the majority of the hospital's physicians; the physicians have to be convinced that complying with measures is good medical care. Today, because data are consistently published, it is clear who is doing better than others. The value associated with evidence-based measures is hard to argue with. When measures are used to evaluate care, resentment over compliance decreases because the measures set an entirely objective standard.

Measures have an additional value in that administrators who use them become in effect part of the caregiving team because they know, for example, that antibiotics are supposed to be given to patients with pneumonia or that infection may be caused by poor hygiene. With measures, leadership has the tools to respond to the community and to meaningfully encourage improvements.

Accountability is promoted when a health care organization uses measurements, because

- Leadership can evaluate the delivery of care.
- Patient care can be evaluated in the aggregate.
- Physicians can be held to an objective standard.
- Nonclinical staff can understand their role in the process of care.

- Leadership can objectively explain financial and resource allocation to the governing body.
- Gaps in patient safety can be identified, corrected, and monitored for improvement.

Things to Think About

A patient in your hospital was placed in restraints due to agitation and to prevent her from harming herself or others. During normal morning rounds, a nurse discovered the patient dead in her bed.

- As an administrator, what do you do?
- How do you handle the media?
- Whom do you go to for information?
- What kind of information do you want?
- What major categories would you anticipate would be involved in the root cause analysis?
- What factors do you think might have contributed to this adverse event?
- How would you develop a corrective action?

CHAPTER SIX

The Rationale for External Drivers of Quality

M y experience when teaching health care leaders about measurements is that they are surprisingly unfamiliar with the pressures that exist in their own business. They find it hard to take in that health care is as much about clinical measurements as about clinical care and that it is measurements that are driving changed practices and reimbursement. Politicians speak about health care problems and suggest reforms because they want to respond to public pressure to improve hospital safety, to experience excellent evidence-based medical quality, and to have better coverage for insurance. Health care is news; everyone needs it, and it is extraordinarily expensive. Together, the public and its representatives, the politicians, are hoping to make an impact on the industry. And they are in fact changing health care in the United States. The government is so involved in what is primarily individuals' personal business because the public pressures its representatives to be involved and to monitor the industry and to improve it.

In this chapter I will discuss how governmental regulations have an impact on the health care industry and how private business and community groups are dictating hospital standards as well. I will also outline how quality management departments can be used to mediate between the health care organizations and these external drivers of quality care.

THE GOVERNMENT TAKES THE LEAD

The federal government, and also to some extent state governments, has a lot to say about the public's health. Business patrons are forbidden to smoke in public places; women are advised to avoid alcohol when pregnant; children are required to receive specific vaccinations before being admitted to public schools; all of us are asked to heed the nutritional standards recommended by the government; and the media write constantly about health care issues from obesity to autism.

The government monitors health care through data derived from research and statistical information posted by various agencies and professional societies. The media, in turn, translate the statistics for the nonprofessional community and interpret the data in relation to lifestyle and survival. In addition to informing the public about health care issues, the government has taken on the responsibility of monitoring hospital care. Hospitals and health care organizations are now required to collect data on defined indicators of care, and the government is offering financial rewards if that care conforms to what it defines as the standard of care. If hospitals don't conform to these indicators or measures of quality care, they run the risk of losing government reimbursement. The government insists, for example, that patients diagnosed with heart failure should receive education about the importance of monitoring their weight and that patients with pneumonia should receive education about smoking cessation. It doesn't take a great leap of imagination to see that today the government has effectively taken over the role traditionally reserved for the physician—dictating patient care.

MONITORING QUALITY
FOR CHANGED PRACTICES

Because the public is so adamant about its desire for safe health care, the government is trying to reform the highly individualized (and antiquated) health care culture in which the individual physician is rarely questioned and poor outcomes are thought to be a necessary correlate to disease. If their organizations are to succeed, or even to survive, health care administrators and others responsible for formulating policy need to understand the health care forces active today and the processes that have developed. External forces, such as those shown in Figure 6.1, are shaping health care priorities, and hospitals have to respond.

A brief summary of the history of monitoring quality reveals how the interrelationships among the patient, the physician, the health care organization, and external forces, such as the government and business, have changed. From classical times, when physicians pledged through the Hippocratic Oath to "do no harm" to their patients, to today, methods of monitoring patient harm and maintaining safety have changed dramatically.

For many centuries people thought of the art, almost the magic, of the physician as healer. Then the application of the scientific method and statistics in the nineteenth century helped clinicians relate cause to effect through observation and interpretation of data. Florence Nightingale is among those credited with promoting the value of performing statistical analysis on aggregated patient data to discern meaningful patterns linking processes and outcomes. In the twentieth

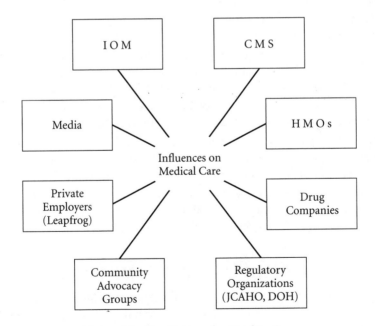

Figure 6.1. Key Drivers for Quality Care.

century, with the rise of theories of standardization applied to maintain quality control in industry, health care services began to be monitored through organizational processes, and health care organizations, rather than specific physicians, were scrutinized by the government (through the Joint Commission on Accreditation of Healthcare Organizations) to ensure that appropriate standards of care were being met.

Quality theorists began to formulate methods and methodologies to approach zero defects in various products, and the idea of analyzing structures and processes to standardize outcomes took root. In the past few decades the government and private agencies have begun to monitor health care quality by imposing standards that have to be met not only for accreditation but for financial incentives as well. Safety has been interpreted by these agencies as literally measuring up to a preestablished standard of care. Data are expected to be collected, aggregated, analyzed, and reported to the government and to the public.

The era of accountability is taking hold. External forces require hospitals and care providers to make clinical decisions that may not be the same as physicians' traditional practice but that are based on aggregated evidence. Individuals responsible for overseeing hospitals should involve themselves in understanding variation from the gold standard of care (evidence-based medicine) and should require accountability from staff about any variation from established standards.

When physicians and nurses complain about how much paperwork is required by external agencies to document the delivery of care, they fail to recognize that documentation is communication and that lack of documentation is poor communication and often reflects poor care. The complex health issues of patients require many pieces of data and various experts to analyze that information in order to arrive at the proper diagnosis and treatment. This complexity is compounded by the fact that individual clinicians take care of many patients in a short period of time. No one can remember everything. Physicians, managers, administrators, and directors of ancillary services need to analyze not a single patient but all the patients under their supervision. Without accurate records, mistakes happen.

THE MEDIA CARRY THE MESSAGE

In a recent conversation with a journalist from *Newsday* (a local Long Island, New York, newspaper) about hospital quality data that had been published, I realized that she had more impact on quality management than I did. When she published data on treating AMI (acute myocardial infarction, or heart attack) patients with aspirin on arrival at the hospital, the governing body of our system, together with hospital administrators, took notice and determined to make improvements in the cardiac program a priority. They directed me to work with the clinical staff to improve the delivery of care to this patient population. This reaction was the result of the pressure that *Newsday* readers exerted on the health system by calling members of the board of trustees and administration asking for clarification on the published results. I don't think an internal report of quality management data would have evoked the same energetic response.

The media are very powerful. Good results revealed in a quality management report may not much impress the administration, but good results published in the *New York Times* are a cause for celebration by leadership. Good publicity is good for business. I was once sitting in the lobby of a community hospital when a member of the community walked in and asked to speak to an administrator about a recent article in the *Times* about this hospital being the "best hospital." He said that he had just left another hospital where he was being treated because he wanted to come to the best. Good publicity draws patients into the hospital; increasing patient volume improves the financial situation of the hospital.

Because the public reacts to the health care numbers that are interpreted by the media, hospitals have to react as well. Therefore hospital leaders and administrators and those involved in health care policy have to understand the data that are being collected and publicly reported. They have to respect the concerns of the public. The medical errors that make the news rightfully frighten the public. No one wants to be burned in an MRI machine or have the wrong leg operated on or acquire an infection because of poor sterilization practices. Hospitals have to comply with the indicators of good care set by the Centers for Medicare and Medicaid Services (CMS). They have to understand what insurance companies are looking for as they negotiate contracts for reimbursement. They have to have numbers at their fingertips to respond to the media reports of unsafe practices. "Don't worry," just won't cut it.

Health care leaders are beginning to understand the strength and power of the public's expectations for quality oversight and the corresponding political, governmental, and media response to those expectations. Patients will go to those institutions that are responsive to their needs and concerns. Hospitals that don't meet the government's expectations will receive less reimbursement or not be accredited; they will fail, economically, socially, and clinically. Health care leaders need to embrace the measurements of this new world of medical quality care by working to support the public's desire for information about services, operations, and policies.

PUBLIC PRESSURE FORCES CHANGE

Public pressure influences more than governmental politics. Private insurance companies are also dictating specific care practices. They too require measurements and indicator data to help them evaluate the product they are purchasing. Health maintenance organizations (HMOs) negotiate contracts with health care organizations, and the rates are more or less favorable depending on how the contracting hospitals manage their product. The HMOs want to know what their dollar is buying, and therefore they require information about processes, techniques, services, and outcomes. They want to get the biggest bang for their buck; a bad product is very costly. Therefore they compare one institution with another, and the only way to compare is through the data, by the numbers. Patient volume, mortality rate, length of stay (LOS), malpractice claims—all these and much more can be compared through numbers. Data show whether the recommended guidelines are being followed and whether resources are being spent appropriately. For example, when a hospital can show through measures that it has a low mortality rate for a cardiac procedure, has few complications, is able to maintain a short LOS for the procedure, has very few patients on ventilators, and so on, it has proved that it can produce a return on the health care dollar investment.

Private coalitions of health care purchasers, such as the Leapfrog Group, define for their participants the measures by which hospitals are evaluated. On the basis of these measures, Leapfrog recommends to its corporate members how to spend nearly $67 billion each year on health care benefits for approximately 36 million Americans. These measures are quite specific. For example, one of the Leapfrog Group's standards is that ICUs should be staffed with full-time intensivists, and Leapfrog recommends that its members' employees choose hospitals with full-time coverage. Leapfrog also recommends that they choose hospitals that perform a high volume of whatever procedure the patient requires, suggesting that practice makes perfect. Another recommendation is to choose hospitals that use a computer physician order entry (CPOE) system to order medications; this is an effort to avoid the medication errors that result from illegible handwritten prescriptions and decimal point errors. The CPOE is an electronic prescribing system that is supposed to intercept potential conflicts in medication orders by checking for patient allergies, possible drug interactions, and correct dosages.

However, these systems are very expensive and require other computerized databases in order to effectively interrelate electronic information. To benefit from a CPOE system, a health care organization has to have a sophisticated information technology infrastructure, with research analysts available to program information and develop databases. The clinical staff has to be willing to take the time to be trained in new technology as well. Most hospitals in the United States don't have the financial resources to implement such elaborate programs, so although the Leapfrog Group recommendations may seem responsible, they are not always practical. Yet private groups such as Leapfrog manage enormous sums of health care spending.

These external groups, from governmental regulatory agencies to private health care purchasers, have a tremendous amount of health care policy clout. They determine the measures that are being collected, evaluated, and compared across the country. They demand proof, in the form of numbers, that the care is excellent.

Consumers are also making an impact on the way health care is changing. They review their bills carefully and question why such a (invariably expensive) test was necessary or why a special consultation was ordered. In other words their scrutiny results in a form of oversight for quality. At the time when all medical expenses were paid by insurance companies or the government, perhaps there was less vigilance and inquiry about the bill. But today, patients, the consumers, often have to pay large sums of money themselves, even when they have coverage from insurance, and they want answers about standards of care and priorities.

In response to consumer demands for excellence, the medical record is the database that is researched; therefore the medical record has to be accurate, legible, and complete. Health care organization leaders may have to step in and reinforce the importance of the medical record as the document that reveals the details of an episode of hospitalization. If a patient's physician is not in compliance with a recommended indicator, the patient can and should take issue with the level of care (substandard) received. If a pneumonia patient was not given a timely antibiotic and should have been, and the result was a longer LOS or a complication with added expense, the patient certainly will question the care.

QUALITY AND COMMUNITY RELATIONS

Community advocacy groups can't actually dictate to professionals how to provide care. What they can do is make their needs known and request information about the reasons standards are not being met. Because the community is taking such an interest in health care monitoring, leadership should use the quality management department to mediate between the organization and the community through an explanation of quality indicators and data.

Community groups can also be helpful in improving communication between the lay public and the professional caregivers. Quality management should help laypeople understand hospital care, including how to analyze adverse events and poor outcomes. Some poor outcomes can't be prevented; some can; some shouldn't occur at all. When the organization describes the processes and methods involved in analyzing its performance, the lay public may be reassured that the hospital is working to make its care safe.

Community advocacy groups are slowly redefining the patient's role as that of a consumer who can demand better care and better outcomes. When a problem does arise, today's health care consumers want much more than a simple explanation; they want to be assured that their issues will be resolved and that other patients will not suffer what they have suffered. In my experience, when an error occurs patients want the corrective action explained more than they want an individual physician or nurse to be censured.

Adverse events require explanation, and quality management can help. For example, if there is a fire in the OR and a patient is injured, that negative outcome deserves an explanation. The goal is not to whitewash incompetence or to increase negative perceptions about health care but to have the organization and the community work together to understand underlying causes and create improvements so errors don't reoccur. The quality management department can reassure the public about the way problems like this are handled, that they are taken very seriously and that reports of adverse events and corrective action plans are sent to the department of health (DOH) and JCAHO. The goal is always to understand and to improve.

Quality management can teach community groups about the underlying reasons for errors or failed processes, explaining how the method of analysis is objective and therefore trustworthy. Root cause analysis usually uncovers that errors occur due to very human failings—such as being inattentive or rushed, communicating poorly, or relying on memory rather than documentation—and not to inadequate education or training. Quality management can assure the community that hospitals carefully monitor the delivery of care and that they are serious about implementing improved processes. Through talking to the public openly, and especially educating people about measures and methods of monitoring care, quality management can help the public understand what may otherwise seem to be opaque and impenetrable processes of medical treatment.

Just recently, I saw a newspaper article reporting on "quality of care" by city—a kind of *Consumer Reports* for regional hospital care. The data for the report were based on CMS measures. The hospitals in various cities were compared for compliance with the measures. The idea was to inform the public about where they would be safest if they had specific conditions, where they would be able to get the best treatment for, for example, heart failure or pneumonia. What does it mean to the layperson who reads in the newspaper that it is safer to be treated in a Boston hospital than in one in Nashville? Quality management can educate the public about these measures, describing how to use them and what they reflect about the provision of care. Advocacy groups should encourage communication between the public on the one hand and quality management and the hospital staff on the other.

Community groups can push for change effectively. Grassroots programs generally make an impact. Politicians listen. Organizations respond. If quality management helps community action groups understand a measure that reports, for example, about administering aspirin to AMI patients or giving preventive pneumonia vaccinations to elderly patients, members of the community can question their physicians about reasons for noncompliance. Also, quality management can explain to the community why a CPOE may be unnecessary and how quality controls to avoid medication errors are in place through the hospital's quality structure.

Measures reflect what people demand: a safe environment, respectful care for the elderly, fail-safes against unnecessary errors, processes of oversight, and so forth. Often patients are loath to complain or even to assert their right to good care. Advocacy groups serve as voices for timid patients, becoming powerful partners with them to insist on improvements.

TRUTH OR CONSEQUENCES

For health care organizations to survive they have to learn to respect and respond to community action groups and to collaborate with them to improve. Especially as measures are reported in the media, the community should be provided with explanations about how to interpret the data and the rankings. When adverse events are reported, the community should understand the process by which the causes are analyzed and the protections implemented to increase safety. Good communication results in improvements. People want to know and understand; they do not want an administrator to say that the data are flawed and therefore should not be taken seriously. The public takes the data very seriously indeed.

When there are problems, the lawyers, afraid of malpractice suits, might recommend that physicians and administrators not talk to the patients or their families. This adversarial climate does not inspire trust. Research shows that it is better for quality and risk management to work together to uncover the reasons for a poor outcome and then to truthfully and openly communicate to the family, to admit to an error or a lapse in judgment if that was the case, rather than bluster on and attempt to obfuscate the facts. If the care was incompetent or substandard, then the hospital should pay damages. However, there are also times when the care is absolutely standard, and still the outcome isn't positive.

I recall one family that was suing a hospital because the elderly father died. Before having necessary cardiac surgery he was well. After the surgery he was dead. The family thought that he had had bad care. When the case was analyzed, it was clear that the care had been up to the standard. The informed consent had clearly and explicitly explained the risks of dying from the procedure, and the patient and family had been informed about how a minuscule and undetectable piece of plaque could cause death. Not everything can be controlled, even with the best doctors providing the best care. When the family and the physicians discussed what had gone wrong, honestly and openly, without any attempt at covering up or making excuses but with genuine sympathy, the family felt better and decided to drop the malpractice suit. Quality management data can also help in such situations by providing explanations about how rarely such events occur and what methods are in place to reduce risks. Quality management data and methods may serve as a way of "keeping a cool head" in a crisis. Quality management collects facts that demystify the complexity of care.

Only a truthful and complete analysis of the facts can explain adverse outcomes. Because JCAHO has recommended that patients and families have an opportunity to be active participants in their care, it might be useful for community groups to attend meetings with the professionals who do the root cause analyses for events, as a means of educating these groups.

QUALITY DATA FORCE CHANGE

Clearly, health care is a product with social, economic, and political value. External drivers of quality—that is, interventions, processes, and treatments that are dictated not by the physician or the hospital but by the government, private agencies, advocacy groups, and consumer groups—monitor the delivery of care and control the future. If the government is the voice of the people, data are the voice of the health care institution. Administrators would be wise to support and invest in whatever tools they have that prove that good processes lead to good outcomes.

Knowing that the hospital uses quality management measures and methodology can assure the public that appropriate care is provided. An adverse or unexpected outcome can be explained as long as the medical record is complete and illustrates good care. High-risk procedures should be performed according to guidelines and documented fully in the medical record. Unfortunately, many clinicians don't want to enter data or document the chart, perceiving this as a secretarial function rather than the compiling of a legal document showing appropriate care, and they intimidate administrators who are reluctant to enforce accountability.

The recent CMS financial incentive program that rewards hospitals that can prove, through careful collection of quality information, that they are compliant with the standards of evidence-based medicine is but one example of how quality data are being used to compare hospital performance across the nation. The data provide a threshold for understanding what is good and what is not good in the delivery of services.

Everyone wants to know the numbers, but getting the numbers from the medical record can be hard because the record is not structured as a database. Nevertheless, it serves as one. For example, one of the CMS indicators for heart attack (AMI) patients is that unless contraindicated, an AMI patient should receive a beta-blocker within twenty-four hours of admission and be prescribed a beta-blocker upon discharge. To meet the CMS criteria for best practices, the administration and the timing of the beta-blocker must be documented, and the discharge prescription must be documented as well. Smoking cessation and prevention counseling at discharge must be documented for heart failure and AMI patients. Many clinicians don't perceive smoking cessation education as an important variable in the delivery of care for a particular stay in the hospital. (Some of the clinicians smoke themselves.)

In a climate where data are used to evaluate and compare hospitals, making use of the hospital's quality management infrastructure makes very good sense. The quality management department is that branch of the hospital responsible for data definition, collection, and analysis. With data, care can be operationalized and safe practices prioritized. With all the agencies, organizations, forums, and interest groups demanding measures of care, it would be seriously out of touch with the times for health care leaders to speak about health issues without statistical information.

Quality management is also changing, as the health care business expands to meet the needs of the public for reassurance and for information. I am being asked, for example, to help set up academic programs in quality in order to educate business leaders and other professionals, physicians and nurses in particular, about how to use data to make clinical, operational, and financial decisions. For example, when leadership at our system wanted to know where our elderly pneumonia patients went after they were discharged from the hospital, what is referred to as their *discharge disposition,* the quality management department developed a database, collected the relevant information, and reported the results (see Figure 6.2). Posthospital placement has an impact on LOS; relationships with nursing homes or rehabilitation centers can be forged if the data suggest the relationship would be profitable. The discharge database proved extremely

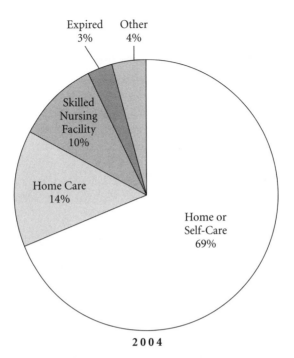

2004

Figure 6.2. Discharge Disposition,
Pneumonia Patients More Than Seventy Years Old.

valuable to the strategic planners in the system. Without these data it would have been difficult to make certain decisions that affect the business of health care.

CASE EXAMPLE: CORONARY ARTERY BYPASS GRAFT

When decisions are not based on data and measurements, they are subjective and rooted in nothing firmer than old habits and opinions. Measures, in contrast, provide a rational approach to analyzing complex interactions of care, personnel, and finance. Moreover, measures require aggregated data; collecting and analyzing these data commit the institution to examining more than an individual physician's practice. More data in, better decisions out.

Consider this example. In 1989, the New York State Department of Health (NYS DOH) began collecting coronary artery bypass graft

(CABG) mortality data provided by thirty hospitals across the state and publishing the results in the newspapers. Starting in 1991, physician-specific mortality data were also collected and published. The state had three goals: to assist hospitals in assessing and improving their appropriateness and quality of care, to help the NYS DOH in its quality improvement activities, and to provide consumers with information that would help them select providers. The DOH developed a statistical risk-adjustment formula model that took into account different patient risk factors and weighted them, allowing for valid comparison across different hospitals. The state was trying to respond to the usual physician disclaimer that the reason some patients died was that they were sicker.

Not surprisingly, the public reacted by going to the hospitals whose published mortality rates were comparatively low. The result of this rather sudden and dramatic shifting of the patient population that required the procedure was to overburden one of our excellent hospitals, which was not prepared for the volume and became overwhelmed. The result of the increased patient volume was a serious rise in CABG mortality; the health system's published ranking changed from seventeenth out of thirty to twenty-seventh. This eventually forced the board of trustees of the hospital to react forcefully, directing the CEO to do something that could ensure good performance. Rather than sending patients to other institutions and so relieving the burden of the extra volume, hospital leadership and the departments of medicine, surgery, and quality management determined to create a better and more efficient system to address patient needs. However, this change of heart took place only after repeated articles in the media identified poor performers.

The power of the pen is indeed mighty. The data the governance group used were the data published in the media. The analysis of the data the governance group used was the interpretation of the journalist. The hospital was not able to criticize the data based on any statistical analysis. The notions that the published data were not accurate or that the hospital's cardiac patients did not fit in the risk-adjustment model were not acceptable. The governance group legitimized the methodology of quality management by assigning to that department the challenge of solving the problem and providing ongoing feedback to that department. With organizational leadership behind this initiative, the CEO offered resources. Technical support flowed into the research division; analysts and data construction specialists were hired.

The first step in the process was to evaluate current practice. A multidisciplinary performance improvement committee was established and guidelines were developed. Surgeons, who rarely concerned themselves with the nonsurgical aspects of a patient's episode of care, were directly involved. The risk-adjusted data from the DOH suggested the survival rate should have been better. When the team reviewed the charts of patients who had died, they concluded that the high rate was due to an influx of sicker, high-risk patients, some of whom had been turned away from other institutions because they were high-risk for mortality. The team then analyzed how cardiac patients flowed through the health system, from the cardiologist's office to postoperative discharge.

Identifying Problems

Problems were quickly identified. Documentation had been inadequate, which resulted in failures of communication. Chart reviews revealed missing data. Practice guidelines had not been developed, and there were no volume requirements in terms of number of surgeries performed for credentialing cardiac surgeons. It also became clear that the existing pattern of crisis management responses to cardiac surgical problems had to give way to a more rational method of proactive guidelines for care, and that a reporting mechanism had to be established so that administrators and the board of trustees could be informed about issues and outcomes.

Case selection also proved to be in need of new policies. Intelligent patient selection requires an evaluation of the appropriateness of surgery, a detailed preoperative workup, estimation of risk, determination of optimal timing, and a formal mechanism for evaluating the surgery's risk-benefit ratio. Our hospital was admitting patients on a kind of *last-resort* policy; anyone who had the slightest chance of benefit would be admitted. Other problems were also revealed, such as a lack of efficient triage. Cardiologists of extremely high-risk patients went surgeon shopping, and surgeons were sometimes called in who were inexperienced.

Although there was discussion of intraoperative problems (such as bleeding) at surgical mortality and morbidity conferences, there was no established format for multidisciplinary analysis and solution of problems. Therefore there was no process to effectively formulate and evaluate policy changes, which is especially difficult across departments.

The surgical ICU (SICU) housed all surgical critical care patients as well as open-heart patients, and there were problems with cross-contamination and sepsis. There was an inadequate supervisory staff. Surgeons and cardiologists, nominally responsible, were often in the operating rooms, in the cardiac catheterization labs, or in their offices, leaving interns, residents, and nurses to identify and communicate problems to the attending physicians. There was also a mixed surgical step-down unit, with much of the same population and problems as in the SICU. When this unit was eliminated during a construction project, cardiac surgery patients were put on a mixed surgical floor with no intermediate care. The result was that cardiac patients were kept longer in the SICU, exposing them to a greater risk of infection, decreased mobility, and a longer length of stay. The staff on the mixed surgical floor were not specifically trained to deal with cardiac patients, and telemetry equipment needed to be ordered and monitored by trained technicians. Again, these conditions led physicians to keep their patients in the SICU longer, and there were readmissions to the SICU from the floor.

Developing Solutions

The multidisciplinary team investigated best practices throughout the country and determined to adopt a formal structure for the heart program, with an administrator to coordinate services across departmental lines. Meetings were scheduled with the multidisciplinary care group (performance improvement committee members and the chiefs of cardiothoracic surgery, cardiology, and pediatric cardiology) and administrative leadership in order to communicate with key hospital decision makers directly. Improved documentation standards were developed for increased accountability and improved communication. Volume requirements were established to prevent the occasional operator from leading the cardiac surgery team.

Practice guidelines were developed for CABGs and valve replacements, based on national guidelines and local expertise. Clinical guidelines were developed with the direct participation of the surgeons to help define and standardize the continuum of cardiac surgical care. All open-heart surgery patients were required to have a cardiology evaluation and clearance, noted in the medical record. This documentation was especially important because patients were often transferred from other hospitals for the procedure, and many did not have an attending cardiologist's evaluation. High-risk patients were evaluated by a multidisciplinary team, ending the practice of surgeon shopping, because the team members had to reach a consensus.

A medical intensivist was recruited as director of a dedicated cardiothoracic intensive care unit (CICU), with complete triage authority. After a year five more intensivists were hired. Since then the CICU has had coverage 24/7 by an intensivist, improving the consistency of postoperative care. The intensivists facilitate improved communication by filling the role of liaison among the patient, the surgeon, the cardiologists, and the internists and other consultants. A staff manual was created for the health care team, covering policies, procedures, and practice guidelines for cardiology patients. The staff manual is regularly updated and functions as an excellent teaching tool for surgical residents and others. It also clarifies what is expected in terms of lines of communication, authority, and accountability. Many other improvements were implemented, including monitoring the timeliness of aspirin administration and establishing a specialized cardiac care unit.

Results of this careful performance improvement program have been impressive. Risk-adjusted mortality among CABG patients has been dramatically reduced. In 1994, the program was ranked fifth in risk-adjusted mortality out of thirty-one cardiac surgery programs. Complication rates were also significantly lower for stroke and sepsis. Patient satisfaction surveys revealed higher patient satisfaction with all aspects of the cardiac services program. Low mortality rates have remained stable despite dramatically increased volume, changes in personnel, and the willingness to accept high-risk patients. The most important reason for the elimination of infection in the CABG population was the establishment of the fully dedicated cardiac unit, staffed with around-the-clock intensivists. For several years there have been no cases of sepsis in the almost 2,300 CABG patients treated during that time.

These process changes and the willingness to openly examine old practices were critical to the improvement effort, as was multidisciplinary communication and discussion of complex issues. But it should be noted that the impetus for the improvement effort was data collected and reported by an external agency. The redesigned cardiology program has reached the forefront of excellence and cost-effective care in the state, despite intense regional competition and public scrutiny.

The point here is that outcomes analysis, when properly applied to health care organizations, improves care and saves lives. Also, by reducing excess expenditures related to complications from less-than-optimal care, health care organizations reduce costs while improving quality of care, even for the oldest and sickest patients. Increasing the public scrutiny of medical outcomes forced this change and resulted in better quality and cost efficiency.

MAKE THE REGULATIONS WORK FOR YOU

Most organizations work from a set of regulations or articulated standards. Working with standards can be thought of as quantifying norms of behavior. This is the beginning of using measures. In order to study or document the level of compliance with any regulation, someone has to define which aspects of the standard are being counted, how much or how many are in compliance, and how many are not. Once calculated, the data have to be evaluated to be meaningful. Monitoring compliance forces organizations to develop a structure for measuring. The JCAHO regulations require such a structure and define it explicitly. There is a definition for everything, including the role of governance, the competency of the staff, the safety of the environment, and the rights of the patient—to name just a few of the arenas JCAHO monitors. For example, JCAHO requires that there be bylaws for the medical staff; if there are, then the organization is compliant with that regulation. But a more sophisticated understanding of the JCAHO requirements is not about compliance but about realizing that the standards define what kind of organization a hospital should be.

The attitude of the CEO and the senior leadership determines the value of the standards to the organization. The standards can be defined as a nuisance, something compelled by an external agency that has to be given lip service every couple of years to get accreditation in order to get reimbursement, but really only an annoyance. Or the measures of compliance can be used as a springboard to quantify the clinical experience, from the physician's office through home care. The standards suggest the most basic framework, but if used properly they can offer administrators enormous help in understanding their organization. Administrative goals and quality goals are entirely congruent, as long as the CEO sees them this way.

JCAHO developed its standards in collaboration with national experts to define the standards of care, the different components of the organization, and the processes of care that relate to the components. Quality management departments are required by JCAHO, to ensure that standards be met, data collected and analyzed, and improvements documented. Unlike other industries, health care is not closely associated with quality control or inspections of its products.

Care issues are extremely complex and require serious analyses—not only statistical analyses but also social and political responses. For example, the measure "infection rate" encompasses many variables. Administrators have to understand the complexity while they are caught in the political and social conflict of opposing forces: the public demands zero infection; the physicians believe this is not possible. This is another area where quality management can be useful; data and measures can be brought to bear in negotiating these issues for administrators. Administrators are caught between the public's pressure and seek to "do something," often without understanding the dimensions of the problem.

When the leadership of our health system made understanding and reducing sternal wound infections a priority, quality management collaborated with physicians to do a careful study of the processes of care. The goal was to define the organism responsible and institute corrective actions and preventive policies. Measures were developed to help explain the phenomenon, tracking rate, type, and severity of outcome. Quality management provided the administration with detailed root cause analyses, a research infrastructure, and databases for analyses. This is a more appropriate application of quality management techniques, which previously were used only to deal with utilization issues, LOS, and accreditation surveys and also for communicating with state and other external agencies.

SUMMARY

External drivers of quality influence health care because

- Political pressure is forcing hospitals to measure specific aspects of the delivery of care.
- The government and private agencies are offering financial incentives for complying with specific standards.
- The public is holding physicians and hospitals accountable for good care.

- The media are publicly reporting quality measures, including hospital- and physician-specific data.
- Insurers of health care services insist on quality measures to ensure a quality product.
- Publicly reported data about unsafe practices provoke improvement efforts.

Things to Think About

The local community newspaper reports that the hospital with which you are associated has a high mortality rate for orthopedic surgery, higher than the rate for comparable hospitals in the state. Your supervisor asks you to look into this issue.

- How would you handle the press and community relations?
- What questions would you ask, and of whom?
- Where would you find information (data) that would be relevant and reliable?
- Which members of the staff would you involve?
- What processes would you use to investigate the situation?
- Whom would you hold accountable for providing you with information?
- What improvements would you implement?
- How would you ensure continued improvement?

CHAPTER SEVEN

Integrating Data for Operational Success

$\mathbb{T}$oday's methods of reimbursement by the government and by health maintenance organizations (HMOs) have compelled senior leadership of health care organizations to focus on key operational variables in planning their organizations' budgets. With the help of the finance department, leadership has come to understand that information about length of stay (LOS), patient throughput, discharge disposition, admission criteria, operating room (OR) turnaround time, and resource consumption has critical financial implications.

Therefore the CEO and senior administrators need to monitor these variables in order to maintain a reasonable budget. Typically, the chief financial officer, through the budget process, reports on these operational and clinical variables without reference to the specifics of patient care or of quality. Quality is considered to be separate from a sound budget, but this distinction between financial and quality information makes it difficult for leadership to identify problems and improve hospital operations. Ideally, the quality management department should provide reports of clinical and operational variables that combine with financial reports to produce the hospital's budget. A combined report would be especially useful because the government requires hospitals to report quality data for accreditation and higher reimbursement.

In this chapter I will offer examples that reinforce the relationship between maintaining quality standards and gaining operational and financial efficiencies. I will illustrate that when leadership is committed to improving quality, and uses measures and quality data to monitor processes and develop improvements, the organization benefits financially.

DIFFERENT DATA TELL DIFFERENT STORIES ABOUT CARE

Report cards are one useful way to translate the experiences of individual patients into a collective representation of the delivery of care. With the aggregated data of report cards, analysis can move from patients' responses to the question, "How do you feel?" to information about the probability of recovering from a specific procedure or disease in comparison to a similar patient at a comparable institution. That's a big leap. The report card reflects what it means to have specific treatments at particular places.

Report cards compare hospitals; they force organizations to measure themselves against other similar organizations and against a gold standard (evidence-based medicine). Administrators should take the data from these report cards very seriously and use this information to communicate with the medical staff. Together, administrators and clinical staff can figure out why the data reflect what they do. If the data show that outcomes are poor for certain procedures, administrators should ask the clinicians to examine their processes and explain what led to the poor results. When the administrative approach is analytical rather than confrontational, processes can be examined and improved.

Individuals involved with public health and health care administration should examine the different kinds of report cards so that they can evaluate them. To properly evaluate report card information and use it effectively, administrators should know the source of the data, the reason for the collection, and the intended audience.

WORKING WITH ADMINISTRATIVE DATA

Health care administrative data are readily available, a matter of public record. Because these data are collected for financial reimbursement, they are descriptive, revealing what was done and to whom, but not how or why. It is precisely because these data are administrative that physicians tend to ignore the reports that are generated from them. They know that the data are not subtle enough to accurately represent clinical care.

Physicians often express reluctance to use administrative data to change practice because these data are derived from billing forms, which may not accurately reflect severity of illness or comorbidities and which are entered by clerical personnel, of varying skill, who lack clinical knowledge for interpreting the significance of various diagnoses. It is, for example, difficult to differentiate from the database between comorbidities that might have helped precipitate a stroke (pneumonia or acute myocardial infarction) and those that might have been a complication of the stroke. The only outcome in administrative data is death or survival. However, even if the measure is invalid, when it gets published that your hospital has the highest mortality or infection or complication rate in the state for a specific diagnosis or procedure, it may reveal some problem about the delivery of care. Certainly, such a report will create a public relations issue.

Administrative data, because not clinically motivated, can be insensitive to important aspects of hospital care. For example, if a small community hospital does not have the capability to perform complex cardiac procedures, such as cardiac catheterizations, patients who require those procedures are transferred to a hospital that is equipped to perform those procedures. However, those patients who are inappropriate for transfer because they are too ill or are in the end-of-life stage of care remain at the small hospital. Therefore, when administrative data are collected, it appears as if the community hospital has a very high mortality rate for cardiac patients, with the implication that the hospital is providing very poor care. The actual situation cannot be captured by these data.

In this particular case those hospitals that were receiving very poor report cards due to this problem complained, and the model was changed to account for patient transfers. Unsurprisingly, when the model changed, the results changed. Unfortunately, once a hospital is labeled as "bad," it is difficult for it to say that the data are wrong. Even if methodologically flawed, the public who read the reports don't realize it and react.

Large purchasers of health insurance, such as General Electric and Ford Motor Company, have access to hospitals' administrative data and hire analysts to develop models from these data to determine the expected mortality for particular diagnoses. The companies then can

compare hospitals. The models contain such demographic information as age, gender, comorbid conditions, geographical region, diagnosis, and outcome (mortality). The analysis can point out that one
hospital has a better performance than another and that the likelihood
of dying at one is a certain percentage higher than it is at another. On
the basis of these data, the companies can recommend hospitals to
their employees. If an employee goes for a procedure and has complications, a long LOS, or an infection or if he or she requires extensive
nursing home care or rehabilitation, it costs the purchaser more
money than more effective and efficient care would. Therefore, even
though these reports are based on administrative data, they have a financial impact on the industry.

WORKING WITH PRIMARY DATA

Primary data, unlike administrative data, are more clinically oriented.
Primary data are recorded by physicians and nurses, not by financial
coders. When primary data are coupled with evidence-based medicine, the resulting information can be used to examine the cause and
effect relationship between treatment and outcome. This relationship
is critical for administrators and business leaders to understand. From
a business point of view, understanding the profitability of certain
procedures and operations can lead to increasing the profit margin of
the institution. In order to understand the impact that clinical care
has on institutional operations, it is necessary to examine that care in
the aggregate. Once care can be explained intelligently and objectively,
leadership can take appropriate steps to create a suitable environment
and to develop rational, data-driven approaches to care. Once leadership understands the care delivered at the institution, resources can
be spent more appropriately.

If data are to be used to improve care, then these data should be
primary, collected for the express purpose of understanding the delivery of care. When working with administrative data, you can correlate variables from the database, but when working with primary
data, you can actually make certain assumptions and collect data that
confirm or deny those assumptions.

For example, the State of New York began collecting primary data
with the objective of building a scientific report card that could be refined over time and respond to new information. By collecting primary
data about specific diseases, the state forced clinicians to document specific data points in the medical record. From this information a model

was developed by a task force of experts from around the state that attempted to explain why people died, not simply encode that they did die. Unlike the secondary data from the administrative databases, this model had some explanatory power.

Report cards, ideally, should be used to discover what can be done to improve care and to evaluate the impact of particular treatments on outcomes. Unlike administrative data, which are not suited to analyzing medical practice, the data from the Centers for Medicare and Medicaid Services (CMS) can pinpoint the population the CMS wishes to study and whose health the agency wants to improve. Analysts determine the specific population and set elaborate exclusion criteria so that the population can be reliably compared. For example, people who suffer heart attacks have all kinds of other issues. One instance of this is that research shows that people who are on dialysis and who require a coronary artery bypass graft (CABG) have a greater risk of dying than other CABG patients do. Therefore, in studies of cardiac mortality among CABG patients, recently dialyzed patients are excluded from the mortality data. This is one of the great advantages of using primary data—the measures can be revised and refined as information leads to increased knowledge.

The CMS uses primary data to assess and improve care; the core measures reflect the assumptions that were made. The assumptions are not plucked from thin air, of course, but based on the evidence of experts and on research.

CASE EXAMPLE: STROKE

Stroke is estimated to affect three-quarters of a million Americans annually and is the third leading cause of death in the United States. Research has not compelled specific treatments for stroke, and therefore there is tremendous variability in how stroke patients are managed. Administrative data are used by external drivers of quality to rank hospitals according to outcomes for stroke. Hospitals with poor outcomes protest the shortcomings of the administrative databases and express the feeling that even the risk-adjusted data cannot possibly address the differences in patient populations among hospitals.

However, administrative data can provoke a useful discussion about care. At one of the hospitals in our health system, risk-adjusted stroke mortality was publicly reported to be higher than the rate found in the rest of the state over a four-year period. The appropriate question to ask when confronted with such data year after year is why? Without the aggregated external data, no single physician or administrator would even have known that mortality was high, never mind inquiring into the cause. When asked about the poor ratings, the physicians said that stroke patients are often elderly and very sick and that dying is a normal consequence of the illness. Perhaps it was possible that this hospital's patient population was consistently sicker than the population at other hospitals, but even with that assumption care processes could be examined. If this assumption were correct, we should have been able to verify it easily by examining the medical records (primary data) of those elderly patients with stroke who died. Which is exactly what we did.

A multidisciplinary committee analyzed administrative data from nine health system hospitals that admitted a significant number of stroke patients each year, and created a statistical model similar to the approach used in establishing hospital ratings. Our quality management department maintains a database for all system hospitals. For each patient discharged the data include the diagnosis (or more precisely, diagnosis related group, or DRG), ICD-9 codes for comorbidities and complications, various procedure codes, and demographic information. This database allows the physician to review his or her patient population at a glance.

The CMS and two other governmental departments, the National Center for Health Statistics (NCHS) and the Department of Health and Human Services, have set guidelines for classifying and coding health status according to diagnosis and procedure using the International Classification of Diseases, 9th Revision, often referred to as the ICD-9 codes. These guidelines for coding have been approved by the American Hospital Association, American Health Information Management Association, CMS, and NCHS. The goal of the coding guidelines is to maintain consistency and completeness in the medical record.

A regression procedure was used to derive a model to predict death based on premorbid factors. This model described a clinical phenomenon that can be used by clinicians to understand their patient population in terms of factors contributing to patient death. An explanation of death per patient is very different from an explanation of death per population. A single death may be interpreted as part of the accepted statistics for the patient's disease, but data analysis of a patient population can provide some clues as to causes and or relationships between complication and death.

Because the departments of neurology and quality management took seriously the administrative data that described stroke mortality as greater at our hospital than at other hospitals across the state, the multidisciplinary committee examined primary data from the medical record as well, in order to delve deeper in the effort to discover the reason for the mortality. The clinicians reviewed a sample of the charts, matching all stroke patients who died to a randomly selected stroke patient from the same hospital from the same year who survived.

The first step was to confirm whether the administrative data were accurate and reliable. When the charts were reviewed by a neurologist to determine if the diagnosis of stroke was appropriate, coding problems were exposed. In one hospital the miscode rate was quite high, and also the mortality among miscoded patients was higher than that among the correctly coded patients, thereby artificially increasing overall mortality for the stroke group. This is an important lesson. Because CMS and insurance companies use such administrative databases to compare hospitals' mortality rates, and for reimbursement, proper coding is important.

Analysis identified seven variables that significantly predicted mortality—age, atrial fibrillation, congestive heart failure, dementia, intracerebral hemorrhage, diabetes mellitus, and anemia—and a formula was developed to calculate the probability of death. The relative risk of death was calculated for each stroke subtype, and then a measure was derived that provided an overall estimate of stroke severity in each hospital in the study.

In examining the medical records of those stroke patients who died, the team noticed that a high percentage had the secondary diagnosis of aspiration pneumonia. Stroke patients typically have trouble eating and swallowing, and the result is that the lungs can be affected. One of the ways to avoid aspiration pneumonia in stroke patients is to give them speech and swallowing therapy. The charts of the patients who died did not indicate that they had that therapy. By looking at the primary data—the medical record—important hypotheses could be made about improving care. The administrative data defined the problem, and the primary data analyzed its cause. The information led to changed practices (increased speech and swallowing therapy) and the mortality rating improved.

After the chart reviews and analysis the data were reviewed with neurologists from all the system hospitals, who agreed to collaborate in an effort to improve outcomes for stroke patients. Mortality was higher in bedridden patients receiving heparin and lower among patients receiving physical therapy, who then had less risk of deep vein thromboses. Blood sugar and blood pressure also were found to be important elements in positive outcomes. Reviewing the data in the aggregate, the group was able to develop consensus regarding an improved and standardized stroke treatment protocol.

OPERATIONAL DECISIONS AND QUALITY DATA

When the data reveal good processes and outcomes, it's good for business. The case mix index (CMI), a number reflecting the complexity of treatment given a patient, is based on several clinical variables. Because the health care institution gets paid more for a higher CMI, financial and administrative departments have become familiar with analyzing case mix. Administrators track these variables over time, identifying the ratio of surgical to medical patients (the institution gets more reimbursement for surgical procedures), just as they track census information, which provides data on how many patients are admitted to and discharged from the hospital. Census information and variables related to CMI have operational implications for administrators. For example, information about how many patients are in the hospital and for what kinds of medical treatment can influence decisions about staffing ratios, space allocation for different departments, and technology purchases. Therefore clinical and financial variables together affect administrative choices about organizational operations.

The budget reflects the financial goals, priorities, and operations of the hospital. The CEO wants the budget to reflect the idea that the hospital is run efficiently and effectively and that patient outcomes are good. Unlike some other industries, there is a very low profit margin in health care. Hospitals can't offer discounts. Regulations have to be followed, and the government controls how much money the institution gets paid. Therefore, expenses need to be monitored very closely and processes analyzed carefully. Administration needs appropriate weapons, in this case, the facts based on data, to explain to the governing body the workings of the hospital and how they have an impact on the profit margin.

The goal for administrators is to establish some criteria by which to judge whether certain investments are worthwhile and how different variables interact and are related to each other. Quality management can explain the process of care by identifying and reporting data on crucial variables that influence profit and loss. With quality data, administrators have tools at their disposal to balance clinical, operational, and budgetary issues.

Compliance with regulatory indicators is only one of the reasons to collect quality data. In addition to the numerical data and rankings released on public report cards, qualitative data are also reported in other forms. The Joint Commission on Accreditation of Healthcare Organizations (JCAHO), for example, publishes a hospital scorecard that describes areas that require improvement. For example, the public may be informed through the JCAHO report that patient assessment at a hospital is poor or that a hospital is using inappropriate and dangerous abbreviations when ordering medication. These data are evaluative. The more areas that "need improvement," the more vulnerable the hospital is to having accreditation problems, because this evaluation suggests poor processes and inadequate facilities, oversight, and operations.

QUALITY AND RISK

Quality management data can help administrators prioritize resource allocation through identifying risk factors in various processes. Quality management methodology analyzes processes proactively, using the failure mode and effects analysis (FMEA), and retrospectively, using root cause analysis (RCA), to find gaps in care that can cause adverse events that are costly from a patient care and organizational point of view. The FMEA, required by the JCAHO as a safety precaution, analyzes the process of care with the goal of identifying the likelihood of a particular process failure and attempts to locate the risk points in a process. Once gaps are found, the multidisciplinary team conducting the analysis estimates the relative harm of that potential error and determines a criticality index, which ranks the most severe consequences of a failure in the process. Together, information about the probability of failure and information about the consequences of failure can guide improvement efforts. The end product of the analysis is an action plan to improve the potential problem.

The close relationship between risk management and quality management can lead to positive relationships between insurance companies and the hospital, because risk management uses quality variables to determine favorable rates in negotiating with insurance companies. Insurance companies are very interested in knowing, prior to giving coverage, how the hospital handles high-risk procedures. Also, having a good quality measure and a good method of root cause analysis can lead to pretrial negotiation that reduces high costs in malpractice cases. Once best practices have been established, staff can be educated about positive clinical outcomes and the associated reduction of malpractice cases. When quality measures are taken into consideration as part of risk-management decisions, the financial results are excellent.

For example, because medication errors are so commonplace, hospitals' insurance rates can be extremely high. In our system we were able to show our insurers that we had a deliberate process to monitor potential gaps in the delivery of care. One of the improvements in the medication delivery process, for instance, was to have nurses perform a read-back of verbal orders, in order to minimize mishearings and misinterpretations. Data showed that nurses were complying with this safety improvement and that due to this preventive process, errors were reduced. Risk management confirmed the improvement efforts with data that showed that malpractice claims for these errors were reduced. Insurers were then confident that our improvement process was deliberate and that the reduced number of errors was not the result of chance but of careful oversight. Premiums were reduced.

Using measurements and quality management methodology creates efficiency and effectiveness. Proactive safety analysis can reduce malpractice claims and illustrate to insurance carriers that the organization has processes and checks and balances to keep patients safe from harm. This is what our system was able to do with the bariatric surgery protocols, and we gained favorable premiums. Insurers saw that our system anticipated problems and was providing solutions and that the organization was doing its utmost to avoid costly harm to patients.

When there are budget problems, finance often considers staff as an expense. But when there is a high case mix and specialized staff are required for care, then a larger staff might improve patient safety through reducing infection, decubiti, falls, errors, and mortality. Staffing then is not an expense but a way to save unnecessary expenditure that result from problems. The intensive care unit (ICU) may need to have a 1:1 patient-to-staff ratio, but also it may not. With quality data available the acuity of patients can be analyzed accurately and the need for staff assessed. Whereas finance may be able to report on staffing as an expense, quality management may be able to explain the relationship between the care provided by staff and the patient outcome.

When administrators make decisions about prioritizing expenses, it is important that they not cut crucial services that might protect patients from harm. It is the most seriously ill and therefore most vulnerable patients who require the most expensive equipment and highest staffing ratios. Complex patient problems require highly technical equipment and monitoring and the very good management that results in a well-coordinated clinical or nonclinical service. When patient safety is compromised, it is very bad for the organization. When patients die unnecessarily, it is expensive. Mortality reviews require resources, and the bad publicity that accompanies poor outcomes reduces patient volume. The administrator has to understand the concept of unnecessary death (death that might have been prevented by, for example, improving processes to reduce or prevent infection) and be aware of the variables that can be monitored to reduce or eliminate such events.

CASE EXAMPLE: FMEA AND BLOOD TRANSFUSIONS

Hospitals monitor blood transfusions carefully because they are high-risk and complex processes and the consequences of an error, such as delivering the wrong blood to the wrong patient, can be serious, even fatal. Because such great harm can occur, if proactive analysis can prevent an incident that is certainly desirable. Blood transfusion errors occur because the process involves multiple steps and many people, departments, and activities. The FMEA identifies and examines every step in the process.

Think of what is involved. A physician determines that a patient requires a transfusion and writes the order. A nurse draws blood from the correct patient and labels the blood sample with the patient's name. Although this is the first step in a complex process, even here errors can and do occur. In one reported instance a nurse drew the blood from the correct patient, but the vial for the sample did not have a label and she put the blood in her pocket for future labeling. Hospital policy dictated that blood must be labeled at the patient's bedside, but this policy was ignored. The nurse got busy, drew blood from another patient, labeled the wrong blood with the wrong name, and an incident occurred. Such a simple thing—not having a label or a pen—can cause a serious problem.

Between the blood draw and the final blood administration there are multiple steps, with each step susceptible to error. Once the blood is drawn and correctly labeled, someone has to transport it to the lab, where the blood has to be accurately analyzed for type and other elements. Once the patient's blood is properly identified, the matching blood for the transfusion is located at the lab and labeled for the appropriate patient. The policy is that someone from the patient's floor is supposed to collect the blood and verify the accuracy of the blood type and the patient. Once the blood is on the floor, the policy is that two clinicians have to verify that indeed the correct blood type is being administered to the correct patient. This is a double verification process to ensure accuracy. However, there are instances when policy is not followed, and one nurse may say she "trusted" the other to do the proper verification. Processes and policies are often not followed to the letter, sometimes with tragic consequences.

Transfusion errors are so devastating and yet so common that JCAHO has communicated some suggestions to help hospitals reduce the risk of making such errors. These suggestions stress developing patient identification policies, perhaps with a unique identification band for transfusions, and double-checking blood verification procedures. They suggest discontinuing the common practice of processing multiple samples at one time, and redesigning the environment so that multiple samples are not stored in the same refrigerator.

Education is essential for policies and procedures to be internalized. When activities become routinized, people can easily shift to shortcuts. However, serious errors are often the consequence of trivial actions. Therefore, stressing conformity to the policies and procedures can save lives, protect patient safety, and improve organizational processes and resource management.

COMMUNICATING QUALITY DATA

Over a ten-year period our quality management department was able to educate key decision makers on the importance of various operational and clinical measures and to establish a matrix of reported data that translated bedside care into operations in a format that leaders could easily view and interpret.

All the measures that are reported out on this high-level quality report (see the sampling in Figure 7.1) have the same intention: to objectively monitor, assess, and improve care and the operation of delivering care. Further, the measures appear in sets that communicate

Outcomes	HosA	HosB	HosC	HosD	HosE
Autopsy request rate	**	*	*	*	***
Excess days per PT	*	*	**	**	**
Unplan 30day readm rate	**	**	**	**	**
Unplan return OR rate	***	***	***	***	***

Patient Safety	HosA	HosB	HosC	HosD	HosE
Nosocomial press. ulcer rate	*	***	*	*	***
PT fall index	**	*	***	*	***
PT red/surg restraint index	***	*	*	*	***
SSI rate	***	**	*	**	***

ED	HosA	HosB	HosC	HosD	HosE
Left AMA rate	*	*	*	**	**
LWBE rate	*	**	**	**	**
Return 72hrs rate	*	*	*	**	***

ICU	HosA	HosB	HosC	HosD	HosE
Mortality rate	*	*	**	*	**
Readm 72hrs rate	*	***	***	***	***
Self-extubation rate	**	***	**	*	***

***/black: Performed BETTER than the benchmark
**/gray: Performed within average
*/white: Performed WORSE than the benchmark

Figure 7.1. Four Examples of the Sets of Measures Reported in an Executive Summary, September 2005.

complex information, increase awareness of problems and successes in the delivery of care, and promote accountability, because care is objectively and continuously monitored over time.

These measures are reported throughout the organization, to the medical boards, the performance improvement committees, the board of trustees, the CEO, and the chief operating officer. A graphic at the top of each set of measures, a small pie chart, conveniently encodes how the organization is doing on that cluster. The measures in Figure 7.1 reflect a great deal of high-level information about various aspects of care. At a glance the sections of the pie charts distinguish whether the reported indicators are better than, the same as, or worse than the established benchmark. Indicators for the high-risk and resource-intensive environments of the emergency department (ED) and ICU are compared across five hospitals. The data show that only one hospital (E) had a good (that is, low) rate of returns to the ED within seventy-two hours. Two hospitals (B, E) showed improved (lower) self-extubation rates. These executive reports enable an administrator to quickly grasp where there are successes and where improvement is needed.

Busy administrators want to get the picture quickly and learn how poor performance can be improved. From this display, leadership can see, for example, that for patient safety measures, the system is doing poorly, with half the pie chart coded white, indicating performance below the established benchmark. With this form of graphic display, a problem needing a solution can be quickly identified.

The goal of communicating data is always to improve, and these and similar measures provide a good starting point for a discussion of how to accomplish this. When multiple hospitals are compared, as we do monthly across our health system, best practices can be identified and shared with others. If one hospital's data show that its pressure ulcer rate is better than the established benchmark (Hospital B or E), for example, it can share its experience with improving the delivery of care with others. Hospitals whose rate is poor, that is, below the benchmark, can ask questions and do a root cause analysis of their processes. These reports are continuous because once improvements are implemented, it is essential to maintain vigilance.

Tracking excess days is a useful quality variable that reflects both efficient and inefficient practices that have a direct impact on the financial health of the organization. Therefore quality management aggregates these data and reports excess days on the executive summary. In order to receive appropriate reimbursement, the organization tries to match the benchmark established by the CMS for specific procedures or diseases. When utilization is appropriate, a low rate of excess days reveals efficiency in the delivery of care. When a high rate of excess days exists for certain procedures, that information may signal a problem, perhaps inefficient processes, problems in communication between different levels of staff or departments, or treatment that resulted in poor outcomes to patients, causing a prolonged and costly LOS. Any noteworthy changes in the data can target a problem area to be investigated, such as discharge planning, delay in treatment, or lack of communication.

When patients must return to the ED within a certain amount of time or make an unplanned return to the OR, resources have to be used that may not be reimbursed, because duplicate procedures are often not insured. When patients in the ED leave without being evaluated (LWBE) or against medical advice (AMA), then the care may not have been efficient. When the surgical site infection (SSI) rate is high, then care processes should be examined. The goal is to balance efficient processes with successful outcomes, and the best way to monitor this balance is through data. The intent of the measures is to capture relevant information that can be clearly illustrated and communicated. Because the measures are reported for specific time periods and tracked over time, problems and improvements can be easily seen. Measures are the best way to objectively assess care or evaluate the performance of caregivers.

From a purely operational point of view, unplanned returns to the OR are a serious problem, one that needs correction. They create a backlog in the OR, which has an impact on efficiency, preventing or delaying normally scheduled procedures. Recovery rooms and other units become taxed as well. When a patient requires a reoperation, insurance companies may feel that there was something wrong with the initial procedure and see it as a quality issue. Clusters of unplanned reoperations, linked either by procedure or physician, should be of particular interest to administrators because they will cost the hospital money and they suggest the existence of a process or competency problem. Only quality management data can provide administrators and leadership with an appropriate and accurate level of oversight. Administrators need to learn to use quality data to understand operations and make decisions.

Consider autopsies. An autopsy provides an accurate diagnosis about the patient's condition and therefore about the physician's accuracy of diagnosis and appropriateness of treatment. Recently, the media reported that several transplant patients died because their organ donor had had rabies, a fact entirely unknown to the physicians. The donor's symptoms were congruent with a drug overdose, and a diagnosis of rabies was never considered. After the patients who received the infected organs died, there was an investigation and autopsies were performed, which is how the rabies was discovered. Autopsies tell the truth. However, there is no reimbursement for the procedure, and organizations don't encourage it. Physicians may be happier thinking they did it right and may not want clear proof that their diagnosis or treatment was incorrect. But by choosing not to know, the organization puts itself in the way of an oncoming error. If there are problems, they are better identified than ignored, but that's a tough position for an administrator to take. This is the reason that regulatory agencies recommend improving organizations' autopsy rate.

Most clinical measures have operational analogues. Administrators can't rely solely on physicians to understand the clinical processes that make an impact on operations. In our system the CEO clearly took the position that all care would be measured, reported, and communicated across the organization. His message was that he was not going to hide from being accountable if there were problems in services. Staff got the message. Measures, that is, the objective evaluation of care, would be used to assess competency. At every level of the organization, measures are used for evaluation and identification of problems, with the clear message that if you don't know what's broke, you can't fix it.

The measures used were not pulled from thin air nor were they imposed on the organization by quality management. The measures were developed over time, with a great deal of multidisciplinary input from various stakeholders who knew the process and the potential for problems. Stakeholders are in a position to understand how measures can make an impact on their work.

For example, as a way to understand the efficiency and effectiveness of the ED, the measure LWBE (left without being evaluated) is collected. Clinicians need to know this measure because they are concerned about providing adequate patient care, and they don't want poor processes. Staff have to be willing to use the measure to evaluate performance. Once that idea is accepted and socialized into the hospital culture, through consensus, the measure becomes an improvement tool, as well as one that promotes accountability. When benchmarks establish the goals for an organization, it is not easy to ignore what looks like poor outcomes. Consistency is also important, and tracking measures over time shows ups and downs that can be addressed. When care is analyzed openly, with the intent to understand and improve, rather than blame and shame, organizations prosper.

CASE EXAMPLE: DECUBITI

Tracking the incidence and severity of decubiti (skin pressure injuries) can function as a managerial tool, one that identifies a defect in the delivery of care. Therefore it is important for the medical board and for administrative and financial leadership to know the rate of pressure ulcers among their patient population and to ensure that treatment is standardized.

Patients with decubiti have a longer than anticipated LOS, and the costs associated with treatment and complications—pain, loss of limbs, infection, and even death—are high. Services related to treating pressure injuries may or may not be reimbursed by insurance. So decubiti should be monitored in the interests of the organization's clinical, operational, and financial success. The decubiti rate can shed light on expenses related to such things as specialty beds, pharmacy (in the form of medicinal products), nursing performance and competence, and staffing ratios. Other operational and clinical issues involve the continuum of care, discharge disposition of patients, communication among staff, and patient outcomes such as sepsis and death.

In our multihospital system, data revealed that the rates of decubiti being reported varied across hospitals and were fluctuating dramatically every month. The lack of consistency made a comparative analysis difficult. One of the issues that the quality management department addressed was the disparity in care at different levels across the continuum. Care practices varied, for example, among the acute care phase of hospitalization, long-term care, and home care. Some patients came to the hospital from nursing homes with preexisting pressure injuries. The challenge was to implement a process that would standardize care wherever the patient interacted with the system, whether on a surgical floor or in a rehabilitation center.

Leadership supported a performance improvement initiative to improve and standardize care throughout the multiple facilities of the health care system. Using the PDCA methodology the quality management department engaged staff in sharing accountability for reducing the decubiti rate by focusing on data collection; the development of clinical guidelines for best practices; educational efforts for nurses, physical therapists, physicians, and nutritionists; and improved communication so that care of patients with decubiti would be standardized.

Quality management staff worked with nursing to develop a single definition that could be used across the system and to establish a method for data collection that would be consistent and valid. This was no easy task and took a year to formulate. There were many issues to be addressed. For example, in assessing the severity of a skin injury, one of the symptoms a nurse evaluates is redness. But how red does the skin have to be to be "red"? Also, in coding the number of injuries, if one patient has three separate skin ulcers, should that be counted as one or three? Until the staff met and started discussing the definition of the measure, these issues had gone largely unaddressed.

To eliminate idiosyncratic judgment our system determined to adopt and make use of an objective scale that gives clear guidelines on how to evaluate the severity of the injury. The scale was adopted for uniformity and completeness of risk assessment, and caregivers were trained in how to use it. It ranks and scores relevant factors that have an impact on pressure injuries, such as the patient's mobility status (from completely limited to no impairment), nutritional status (from very poor to excellent), activity level (from bedfast to frequent walking), and so on. Reddened areas or skin breakdowns are also objectively assessed to determine whether the patient is not at risk or should be placed on the pressure ulcer protocol. Assessment is done daily and as needed to maintain optimal vigilance. However, simply adopting a scale doesn't immediately ensure that it will be used properly, and educational programs were necessary to train the nurses appropriately.

A systemwide performance improvement committee was formed, spearheaded by a collaboration between the quality management and the materials management departments. The committee established guidelines for the prediction of, prevention of, and treatment for pressure injuries. Clinical pathways, called CareMaps, were revised to incorporate skin care protocols. For example, orthopedic patients who may be immobilized are at special risk for pressure injuries; therefore, in the CareMap for total hip replacement, special skin care interventions are listed, including consultations with a nutritionist and physical therapist.

The effort, expense, and time involved in developing appropriate measures were well worth it. Once a single, consistent measure was established, nursing leadership could compare hospitals, and progress could be assessed over time. Education on the decubiti measure helped to focus staff attention on a serious condition that had become somewhat peripheral to treatment. The documentation requirements also served to heighten awareness and improve assessment and treatment. When the system reported data that showed the decubiti rate was reduced, both in volume and severity, the public relations department was able to assure the public that our organization had a decubiti rate well below the national benchmark (see Figure 7.2).

There were other operational and financial benefits to improving care: specialty beds were used more efficiently and medication was streamlined and could be purchased less expensively. The committee discovered a great deal of variability in the skin care products used. Over 160 different products were in use in multiple facilities. Working with materials management staff, the committee streamlined the products to twenty-four, which helped to control costs. A set of performance measures was standardized across the system. These measures recorded whether a risk assessment was documented within twenty-four hours of admission and also recorded the severity and source of injury, topical treatments, and so on. Quality management established databases for reporting the measures, which improved accountability and communication and helped to identify areas of excellence and benchmarks for best practices.

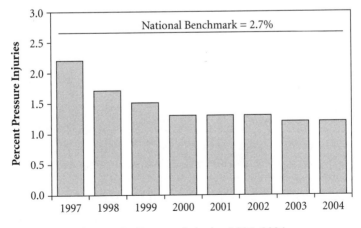

Figure 7.2. Pressure Injuries, 1997–2004.

Quality management defined the methodology that resulted in the decubiti measure; reporting rates and comparing hospitals to a consistent standard helped to motivate action. Hospitals with good rates served as best practice models for those with poorer rates. If the rate of decubiti could be improved at one institution, the process could be duplicated at others.

The initiative successfully reduced the incidence and severity of pressure injuries across the system. LOS was also reduced. Due to the collaboration between quality management and materials management, there were purchasing benefits to the system, with a 24 percent cost reduction in specialty beds and skin care products. Products are now purchased based on quality standards rather than cost effectiveness alone. By standardizing the approach to assessment and by using clinical guidelines, standard definitions, and uniform tools, treatment methodologies, and products, the health system has reduced skin injuries and the expenses associated with them.

MEASURES TELL THE TRUTH

The dilemma facing every administrator is how much he or she wants to reveal about the truth and how much he or she wants to project a positive face to the community. These forces may be at odds. Quality management methodology leads to the truth; it is not a way to gloss over problems but rather to identify and improve them. It is precisely this issue of accountability that makes the use of measures so complex. It is hard to argue with the data, even though most often, if the results show poor performance, people react by criticizing the measures rather than their own performance. The ability to accept objective information, especially when it targets areas that require improvements, is a matter of culture. But it is most important not to hide from the facts, even if unpleasant. Administrative leaders need to understand the problems in the care they deliver and make appropriate interventions to correct problems. It is easy to look at poor report cards and criticize the measures used and say they don't accurately reflect the delivery of care. However, if measures are valued as representations of the various aspects of care, they can be used for improvement.

Clinical staff and institutional administrators are frequently defensive when they see poor results on the table of measures. Interestingly, this is not the case for financial measures that reveal problem areas. For some reason, people can accept financial failures, even to the point of declaring bankruptcy, without becoming defensive. But the same people who can say that they are in a financially disastrous state won't say that they have a clinical disaster on their hands. The health care community is sympathetic to financial problems but less so to clinical ones. Perhaps the reason that clinicians have trouble accepting poor performance revealed through measures is that their highest value is to "do no harm." If the data show harm, this is very troubling.

Administrators also have to juggle their responsibilities between assuring the public that the hospital environment is safe for them and admitting to real problems that may result in a crisis. Generally, bad processes and poor outcomes eventually come to the public's attention, and if there is any suggestion that there has been a cover-up about known problems, that doesn't do the institution, or its administration, any favors.

SUMMARY

Quality data should be integrated into operational and financial decisions because these data

- Provide information for long-term strategic planning.
- Reveal information relevant to daily operations.
- Are required by regulatory agencies for accreditation, compliance, and reimbursement.
- Help the organization balance clinical, financial, and operational information.
- Are publicized on the Web and reported through the media.
- Can be used to evaluate and compare hospitals.
- Define "good" care as compliance with evidence-based indicators.
- Help administrators understand reimbursement.
- Help administrators prioritize resource expenditure.
- Relate seemingly unrelated variables and patient outcomes so administrators can better understand operations and expenses.
- Communicate complex information to various interest groups.
- Reflect institutional leadership's values, goals, and philosophy.
- Help staff evaluate their performance, promoting accountability.

- Translate individuals' experiences into an aggregated and collective representation of the delivery of care.
- Draw on different sources, administrative and primary, to reflect important information about both patients and services.

Things to Think About

Your ED is typically overcrowded and busy. Data reveal that although the CMS requires that pneumonia patients receive an antibiotic within four hours of coming to the ED, these patients are receiving antibiotics between six and eight hours after arrival. As the administrator, what can you do?

- How would you analyze the problem? What variables would you examine?
- Which members of the professional staff would you call on to help you analyze and improve the situation? Why those staff and not others?
- Who would be accountable for improvements?
- How would improvements be measured?
- How would the data be reported? Why in one format rather than another?

CHAPTER EIGHT

Internal Drivers
of Quality

$\sim\!\!\sim\!\!\sim$ E xternal agencies use quality data to analyze care in
order to promote improvements through objective measurements.
Drivers of quality within health care organizations have the same
goal—to use quality data to evaluate and improve clinical care. A leadership commitment is critical to establishing a quality culture and to
promoting quality management methodology throughout every level
of care and throughout the hospital or health care organization. Not
only is it necessary for organizational leadership to support quality
methods but physicians and other clinicians also have to be convinced
that quality strategies for performance improvement—such as working in multidisciplinary groups, incorporating evidence-based guidelines into daily practice, communicating through meetings, performing
careful and complete documentation, and analyzing aggregated data
for trends and commonalities—will lead to improved care and a more
productive organization. Improving the quality of care from within the
organization will be reflected in the publicly reported rankings made
by external agencies.

Quality management departments can and should play an integral
role in ensuring that health care professionals use data to analyze and

monitor the delivery of care and to communicate effectively, across the organizational continuum, the results of that analysis. Unfortunately, however, quality management departments are often underused and relegated to merely ensuring compliance with regulatory requirements and mediating between the goals of the health care organization and those of external agencies. Even though quality management has evolved—from primarily monitoring quality assurance to conducting utilization reviews, developing performance improvement projects, and promoting total quality management—this department is still somewhat removed from hospital operations and has had less status and resources than other departments, such as finance or planning.

For hospital administrators, quality management has been primarily associated with issues of hospital accreditation and with the media and public opinion. Physicians and nurses communicated with quality management staff when adverse events occurred or when poor outcomes and reports needed to be filed with regulatory agencies. It is a rare leader who is committed to implementing quality management processes in order to understand and improve clinical, operational, and financial performance, but this is the approach necessary in today's complex health care environment.

There is no formula or magic kit administrators can use to implement quality management methodologies overnight. To incorporate quality management into the daily fabric of a health care system requires

- Convincing the CEO that it is in his or her interest to have a quality organization
- Developing a methodology that includes collecting data and constructing databases
- Convincing private attendings and nursing and other professionals to adopt quality methods
- Providing constant feedback through measurements
- Conducting continuous monitoring of and communication about the standards of quality

In this chapter I will discuss the advantages of using clinical guidelines to incorporate evidence-based medicine standards into the delivery of care and to improve communication among the caregiving staff. Guidelines help the hospital to standardize care, and identifying variation from the established guidelines helps to pinpoint gaps in the delivery of care. Using guidelines also promotes aggregated data collection because patient populations can be monitored. These data can then be reported through the quality management performance improvement structure so that caregivers receive feedback on the success of their services.

USING GUIDELINES TO DRIVE QUALITY

In the health care system with which I am associated, the quality management department works with administrative and clinical leadership toward reaching the goal of providing safe quality care regardless of the point at which the patient interacts with the system, from ambulance emergency medical service (EMS) through home care. The standard of care should be the same, that is, excellent, at every level of the continuum of care. Success in this goal requires oversight of the care delivered at every stage of each episode of illness and hospitalization, and also effective communication among staff and others at different levels of care. Our health system uses clinical guidelines to effectively promote communication across levels of care and to continuously and concurrently monitor patient safety.

Because our health system is committed to promoting patient safety, maximizing the efficiency of care and the proper use of resources, and to financial responsibility, incorporating clinical practice guidelines and clinical pathways based on those guidelines has proved extremely productive for standardizing care and reducing variation across the system. These clinical pathways, called CareMaps, serve as powerful internal drivers of quality care.

National regulatory agencies, such as the Joint Commission on Accreditation of Healthcare Organizations (JCAHO), recommend the use of clinical practice guidelines, either those promulgated by respected professional societies, such as the Agency for Healthcare Research and Quality, or those developed in-house, to improve quality, utilization, and patient education. Guidelines can also improve treatment protocols. Because individual physicians do not have access to large samples of patients or treatment protocols, they are forced to rely on their individual experience and their judgment, one case at a time. Guidelines make evidence from aggregated populations of patients available to the physician. However, the hospital has to overcome two cultural obstacles that lead to resentment: physicians' perception that guidelines force them to do "cookbook" medicine and physicians' and nurses' feeling that documenting care on the medical record is meaningless paperwork that takes time and effort away from real patient care.

The original intent of the CareMaps was to define patient flow and to provide information for monitoring length of stay (LOS). Standardizing care results in appropriate LOS; unanticipated and unexplained variation from the standard of care increases LOS. CareMaps outline expected key interventions and outcomes along a time line for specific disease processes. When a patient is initially diagnosed, he or she is put on the appropriate CareMap (for heart failure or for hip replacement, for example), with the physician noting what should be accomplished in the patient's daily plan of care (see Table 8.1). The CareMaps incorporate evidence-based guidelines as well as physician orders and clinical judgments. Therefore they are tailored to meet the needs of individual patients.

If a patient does not receive an expected intervention, the reason for the omission is documented on the CareMap. For example, if because of some contraindication or comorbid condition a patient with heart failure doesn't receive an electrocardiogram (EKG) or a chest X-ray that is required by the evidence-based treatment guideline, that important information is recorded on the CareMap variance form and thus made available to all the caregivers on the caregiving team. Likewise, if an anticipated outcome (such as adequate oxygen saturation) does not result from a treatment, that is crucial information for the caregivers as well. At the same time, if the patient does not receive the EKG or X-ray, not due to any clinical reason but because of an organizational problem, such as poor communication among caregivers or inadequate documentation, that omission can be immediately rectified because variance from the expected treatment is also monitored and documented on an ongoing basis.

ENSURING THAT THE STANDARD OF CARE IS MET

The reason communication breakdowns occur is that in today's complex health care environment, it not unusual for a patient to have multiple caregivers from various disciplines, caregivers with little coordination for moving through an episode of hospitalization. Oversight and communication are further complicated by the fact that each

	Met	Unmet	Heart Failure Intervention
Day 1 →			Physical therapy
→			Echocardiogram ordered if EF not known
→			Daily weight performed
→			Patient Friendly CareMap given
Day 4 →			If EF is below 40% discharge on ACEI or ARB
→			Patient discharged with Discharge Instruction Sheet and completed Heart Failure–Specific Supplemental Instructions
	Met	Unmet	Heart Failure Outcomes
Day 1 →			Initial weight on nursing admission form
→			If smoker, smoking cessation counseling given
Day 2 →			EF has been documented in medical record as ____% or mild, moderate, or severe dysfunction
→			Patient given an intravenous diuretic
Day 3 →			Patient given an intravenous diuretic
Day 4 →			EF has been documented in medical record as ____% or mild, moderate, or severe dysfunction
→			Patient is on beta-blocker
→			Patient is given completed Discharge and Heart Failure–Specific Supplemental Instructions

Table 8.1. Heart Failure CareMap.

Note: EF: ejection fraction (percentage of blood the heart pumps with one beat); ACEI: angiotensin-converting enzyme inhibitor; ARB: angiotensin receptor blocker.

of the professionals involved in the caregiving process may have a unique style of interacting with other members of the professional staff, and an individual competency with language, communication skills, and information transfer. Without coordinated care at the bedside, and documentation of that care, both the patient and the organization are vulnerable to clinical and financial inefficiencies, with patient safety vulnerable as well. Without adequate communication, there is an increased risk for undesirable outcomes. The evidence-based clinical pathway serves as a methodology to coordinate and standardize the best quality care for a specific disease process and provides a permanent record of the multidisciplinary plan of care and the delivery of that care (see Figure 8.1).

If hospitals are to improve the quality of care delivered to their patients, communication, discussion, data, and interdepartmental collaboration have to become entrenched in the culture. CareMaps are most useful in promoting interdisciplinary communication and accountability because they make documentation centralized and acces-

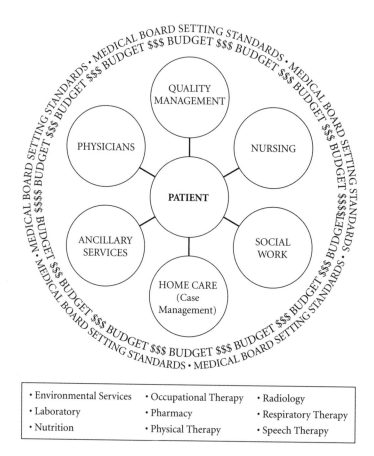

• Environmental Services	• Occupational Therapy	• Radiology
• Laboratory	• Pharmacy	• Respiratory Therapy
• Nutrition	• Physical Therapy	• Speech Therapy

Figure 8.1. Creating Order at the Bedside.

sible. When working with clinical guidelines the entire caregiving team agrees on specific interventions, outcomes, and objectives—and the treatment is documented daily, as is the outcome of that treatment. In this way the CareMaps promote communication among care providers and the rest of the health care community. They detail specific treatments, actual outcomes, and ideal timing. They delineate the daily schedule of activities that affect the patient.

Everyone has to be on the same page in order for patient care to be continuous and effective. The physician orders the therapeutic interventions that should occur; the nurses monitor that these interventions are timely; other disciplines, such as physical therapy and respiratory therapy, can look at the CareMap and easily discern what treatments have already occurred and what remains to be accomplished; in other words, everyone can see where he or she fits into the overall process of care. Most important, during shift changes, where studies show communication gaps are frequent, the oncoming shift can see at a glance the daily progress of the patient.

CAREMAPS PROMOTE STANDARDIZED CARE

CareMaps are an extremely useful tool for helping the nurse improve the delivery of care because they provide a framework for treatment of a particular disease or condition. Generally, it is the nurse who documents the care services delivered daily to the patient. Because it is outlined on a pneumonia CareMap, for example, that unless contraindicated a pneumonia patient should change from IV antibiotics to oral antibiotics on Day 3 of hospitalization, the nurse can anticipate and plan, not only for one patient but for every pneumonia patient. If there are no unanticipated outcomes, changing medication to an oral antibiotic can signal to discharge planning that the patient will be ready to be discharged on Day 5.

Most important, the outcomes for patients treated according to guidelines are generally superior to the outcomes for those who aren't. For example, data on heart failure patients has shown that the patients on clinical pathways that incorporated evidence-based medicine guidelines had a better record of nutrition consultations and timely medication delivery than the comparison group did. Consequently, those patients had more weight gain and were more compliant with dietary restrictions and medication administration. The patients on the

CareMap recovered more quickly and were able to leave the hospital on time and with fewer complications. Clinicians who were made aware of these data recognized the effectiveness of following the guidelines.

Another advantage of incorporating CareMaps into clinical practice is that their use ensures standardization of care across different facilities. Providing a single consistent standard of care, to be applied whether a patient is treated in a tertiary care facility, a nursing home, an EMS ambulance, or a emergency department (ED), requires a deliberate and defined structure. In order to evaluate whether the care is standard or varies from the standard, it is crucial to carefully formulate uniform definitions regarding treatment. The CareMap provides the outline of the standard of care.

Guidelines establish treatment protocols on a proactive basis, improving safety for the patient. Rather than responding to an event with a retrospective analysis of what might have gone wrong with a single patient (as is done in a morbidity and mortality conference), guidelines can improve care for an entire class of patients—patients experiencing pressure injuries, alcohol withdrawal, or stroke, for example. In addition, in these litigious times physicians can protect themselves from lawsuits if they have documented that the standard of care has been met. This is especially useful when there is an adverse event and the mandatory investigation shows evidence that all processes and procedures were entirely appropriate and that best practices were followed along the treatment plan.

If guidelines are in use, establishing processes for optimal care, any deviation from that care can be noted and addressed promptly. With guidelines incorporated into the CareMap, quality management staff can pinpoint which units and physicians are complying with pathway documentation and which are not.

Research reveals that when patients become partners in their own care, results are improved. Each patient in our health care system who is on a CareMap receives a patient friendly version of the CareMap that outlines what will happen, when, and why. Being informed allows each patient to anticipate and understand his or her plan of care. The explanations that are provided for tests and medication help to reduce patient anxiety as well. Patients who understand the rationale behind monitoring their diet or their fluids, for example, have better results than those who have no information provided. In addition, patient education demystifies the medical process because an orderly plan of care is prepared. For example, patients with heart failure receive information about managing their condition that stresses and explains the importance of weight control and diet, and information about when to call the doctor (see Figure 8.2).

VARIANCE DATA HELP DRIVE QUALITY

Clinical pathways outline a treatment algorithm that works to benefit the patient, the physician, and the organization. Any deviation from the standard of care that may influence the quality of care or the patient's

Heart Failure Patient Friendly
Code 311-D

This product is a general guideline and does not
represent a professional care standard governing
provider's obligation to patients.

Heart Failure	If you have heart failure that has caused you to be in the hospital, it probably means that your heart muscle has weakened to the point where it has allowed your body to collect too much fluid, causing difficulty breathing and/or a low energy level.
Tests	You will have chest X-rays, electrocardiograms and/or echocardiograms done. Stress tests, cardiac catheterization and additional tests may also be ordered by your doctor. Your Health Care Team can provide you with education on all the tests. Blood will be taken from you as ordered by your doctor. It usually is necessary to draw blood early in the morning so that the results are available to take care of you throughout the day. Sometimes blood tests are needed several times during the day to best care for you.
Medications	Your medication will be adjusted to improve your heart function and remove the extra fluid. Medicine that removes the extra fluid is called a diuretic (water pill). All medications will be ordered by your doctor. You may also receive medication called ACE-inhibitors and Beta-blockers. These medications are important in protecting your life and decreasing your chance of being rehospitalized. Feel free to question your Health Care Team about these medications. If you are being given a diuretic (water pill), it is important to note if you are urinating soon after taking the medicine and if you are urinating more, less or the same amount as the day before. Please report this to both your nurse and doctor. By giving you the diuretic early in the day, it helps the doctor to know if that day's dose is working.
Diet	The amount of liquid you drink will be limited to decrease the stress on your heart. Your diet will be ordered by your doctor. You may be on a low sodium (salt) low fat or low cholesterol diet. A Registered Dietician is available to talk to you about your diet needs.
Activity	Walking will help you feel better and improve how your heart works. Check with your doctor and nurse before you begin. Please call for help before getting out of bed for the first time if you are feeling unsteady or weak.
Education	We have made a plan that we believe will get you well as quickly and safely as possible. This plan begins early in the morning with a weight check in order to know if you are losing fluid. Ask about your daily weight. You will also be given information about your condition and the medication you are taking by members of the Health Care Team. You will also be taught the importance of weighing yourself every day and writing it down in
Discharge Planning	Your discharge plan will be based on your needs. If you need help with care at home, or were receiving home health care services, please tell your nurse and ask about home care programs available for patients with heart failure. A Social Worker/Case Manager may visit you to talk about discharge planning. The Health Care Team will go over your discharge instructions and answer any questions you or your family may have. If any questions come up after you go home please call your doctor.

Figure 8.2. Patient Friendly Heart Failure CareMap.

outcomes, alter the expected discharge date, or affect the costs of the hospitalization is collected as variance data, with an explanation.

Variance data force the entire caregiving team to focus on expected interventions and outcomes, and patient-specific variance data allow the team to address causes for variation from the standard in a timely way. In our system, variance data from key interventions and outcomes are collected daily, generating immediate feedback about why the patient is not meeting the expected treatment goal.

A scannable variance form is completed by the primary registered nurse and sent to quality management analysts for concurrent review. Caregivers can be alerted to any variation from the standard of care, and if appropriate, corrective action can then be taken. Variance can also serve as a retrospective performance improvement tool. Reports can be aggregated and sorted by source of variance (patient, family, medical discipline, practitioner) and the resulting data can help to identify the effectiveness of treatment interventions and outcomes for a patient population, such as heart failure patients.

Constant feedback is an important element of improving the delivery of care. Retrospective analysis of variance data determines whether or not there are patterns and trends that require improvement efforts. Not only can potential managed care problems be identified through retrospective variance analysis, but payers are more amenable to negotiating favorable contracts when they are confident that a process is in place to quickly identify problems that might result in a prolonged LOS. Again, clinical and financial efficiency are interrelated.

When data reveal gaps in the delivery of care, action can be taken. For example, aggregated data regarding outcomes for pneumonia patients were analyzed for a one-year period and showed that discharge instructions, including smoking cessation counseling, were not being delivered effectively. Improvement efforts were then targeted toward a better process, and care was thus improved for this patient population.

Data are aggregated to identify trends. For example, if congestive heart failure (CHF) patients are not receiving ACE (angiotensin-converting enzyme) inhibitors on the first day, the variance data record why not and also where in the hospital this is happening. The database can analyze care from the system level down to the individual physician. Variance data help leadership prioritize improvement efforts and assist the clinicians with comparative data for education.

Measures, such as the number of days a patient is hospitalized, don't explain *why* a patient had a comparatively short or long LOS.

However, tracking information on a CareMap details the patient experience on a daily basis: what treatments were delivered and what outcomes resulted. Because any variation from the expected algorithm of care is documented on the CareMap, complications are quickly identified and can be treated. Variance data help identify problems during a patient's stay, a result that is especially useful in understanding LOS and evaluating whether care was appropriate.

The use of CareMaps has been shown to have great value. Not only do they create order at the patient's bedside by coordinating and documenting care but they also allow caregivers and administrators to monitor interventions and outcomes for quality as well as for cost and resource effectiveness. Because clinical pathways reinforce multidisciplinary communication, accountability is increased. Everyone involved in managing the patient is conscious of being part of an interdependent team. This patient-centered mind-set works to the advantage of the patient and the organization. The CareMap methodology has helped our system reduce day-to-day variation in resource and treatment patterns and at the same time has provided a framework for building a highly efficient, outcome-focused care delivery system.

DEALING WITH RESISTANCE TO CAREMAPS

Introducing change frequently meets with resistance, and learning to use CareMaps is no exception. Some nurses reject the CareMap as meaningless paperwork; some physicians reject the CareMap as cookie-cutter medicine. Providing education about CareMap value helps the organization at every level. Although some physicians may resist using CareMaps, either because they feel it overrides their autonomy or because they feel it is a nursing tool and does not concern them, others see the advantages. They realize that their individual knowledge coupled with the aggregated knowledge of evidence-based medicine will lead to the best results.

Nursing staff are generally less reluctant than physicians to implement CareMaps but still require education on CareMaps' use and usefulness. To accomplish this in our system, quality management staff went to the different hospitals to establish train-the-trainer programs in individual units so that there would be on-site expertise in how to use the CareMap and fill in the variance form. By examining the CareMap the nurse can see at a glance what treatment or tests were accomplished on a specific day and what the next step in treatment should be, and with what expected outcome. Especially valuable during shift changes, when crucial information regarding individual care plans can be lost, this permanent record of information can help the nurse organize the patient's care. Once a nurse realizes the advantage of CareMap documentation to patient care and to the organization of the unit, his or her reluctance to use it decreases.

IMPLEMENTING GUIDELINES TO DRIVE QUALITY CARE

Guideline development, implementation, and acceptance involve lengthy and complex processes. Multidisciplinary, disease-specific task forces, composed of potential clinical stakeholders from across the organization, should meet to evaluate and develop guidelines that are both based on the literature and individualized to meet the needs of the specific institution. Professional buy-in to guidelines helps to ensure their acceptance. When multidisciplinary teams develop the internal guidelines, research the expert literature, and champion guideline implementation to their peers, consensus for guideline use improves. Using multidisciplinary teams at this stage also increases accountability in treatment because the different disciplines have agreed on what is expected and how to coordinate services. Another advantage to asking the stakeholders to develop the guidelines is that they understand the limitations of the institution, the kinds of implementations that are realistic, and the resources that can be tapped. As with all improvement efforts, administrative leaders must support the task forces and their goals for the improvements to be effective.

In our system, after months of development, guidelines are presented to the appropriate performance improvement coordinating group for discussion and evaluation. Once finalized, the guidelines are reviewed by the department chair or director of the appropriate service, the medical board of the hospital, the nurse executive, and the multidisciplinary quality improvement committee before approval. With so much professional input and so many evaluative opportunities, clinicians feel less as though they have had something imposed on them from an external source and are more willing to use the guidelines.

Once approved, guidelines still have to be continuously monitored for ongoing effectiveness and updated as appropriate. As new information and technology influence medical treatment, guidelines have to be revised accordingly so that patients receive the most current standard of care. Educating the staff about such revisions can take many forms—system and hospital committee meetings, patient care rounds, in-service training programs, teleconferences, and train-the-trainer programs. Through education about the benefits of guideline implementation, administrators and managers help to create a climate where physicians are encouraged to standardize care.

EVERYONE BENEFITS FROM CAREMAPS

In developing disease-specific CareMaps, the goal is to outline appropriate care and the appropriate time frame for that care: what to do, in what order, and by whom. CareMaps allow caregivers to access the treatment plan of every patient and the results of that treatment each day. Also, because the CareMap is forward looking in that it outlines the following day's treatment, organizational efficiency is improved because the nurses know what has been done, what the result was, and what is next in the treatment plan. All information is in one spot, not scattered in notes throughout the patient's chart.

For the physician the CareMap becomes a database, documenting, for example, that aspirin was given on time. For administrators the CareMap provides a tool for understanding and improving patient flow. If all caregivers know what they are supposed to do every day, they can effectively prepare and plan and communicate. Because the measures recorded on the CareMap are also those required by the Centers for Medicare and Medicaid Services (CMS), completed CareMaps help the hospital meet CMS data collection and reporting expectations. The CareMap is also a useful tool for monitoring patient safety. The CareMap can be used as a research tool as well because isolated variables can be extracted from multiple CareMaps and analyzed in the aggregate.

CareMaps improve patient throughput because the outlines of the treatment per diagnosis are in place. Therefore, as soon as a patient is diagnosed in the ED and the appropriate CareMap put in the chart, everyone involved knows what to do and what to expect within a specified time frame. Expectations can be set and predictions can be made. For example, if a stroke is identified in the ambulance by the EMS staff, the ED can prepare the appropriate treatment, all outlined on the CareMap, such as a CT scan and administration of tPA (tissue plasminogen activator) if timely. Used properly, a CareMap produces best practices and promotes critical thinking, always a challenge to maintain in the face of so many routine tasks.

JCAHO has recently introduced *tracer* methodology into its accreditation surveys, because of its concern about gaps in communication and problems with moving the patient through an episode of hospitalization. JCAHO is looking to trace the patient's care from the time of entry to discharge. Today, because multiple caregivers may be involved and different departments and disciplines interact with the patient, it is most important for a hospital to have coordinated communication and coherence in managing care. Nurses are expected to report the entire hospital experience when surveyors question them; the CareMap provides help here because it traces and documents the patient's experience, from diagnosis to treatment to discharge. In addition, the CareMap helps clinicians verbalize the delivery of care to the JCAHO surveyors because it records what happened, which tests were administered, and what results or outcomes ensued. Furthermore, if there was variation from the standard, the explanation is noted directly on the CareMap.

As processes are improved with effective CareMap use, adverse events are also minimized. Research has shown that most serious medical errors are caused by a lack of communication among caregiving staff, a lack of proper assessment of the patient, or a lack of documentation. When caregivers don't know what has occurred in the patient's treatment, it is difficult to avoid mistakes. The CareMap outlines a coherent treatment plan and is useful for designing effective work strategies, maintaining appropriate LOS, improving interorganizational communication, especially shift to shift, and functioning as a diary of past care and a blueprint for future care. CareMaps provide an effective internal driver of quality care.

DOCUMENTING THE DELIVERY OF CARE

A CareMap is more than a checklist because it predicts what will occur each day in the normal course of treatment and provides a record of what has occurred previously. The checklist component of the CareMap reminds the caregiver of what should be accomplished: check the vital signs, administer medication, begin the discharge plan. Then the CareMap goes further by informing the caregiving staff about what should happen every day, and if an outcome does not happen as predicted, the explanation is recorded as variance data. When quality management analyzes the variance data, problems can be located and changes can be recommended based on objective information.

CareMaps, being concurrent documents of the care provided, enable staff to constantly update information. Therefore decisions can be made with a complete background of what was done and when and with what result. Because circumstances change constantly as the patient progresses through the episode of hospitalization, decisions are being made all the time. These decisions, when based on reliable information, such as the CareMap provides, are then grounded in evidence, not in a (perhaps biased) subjective experience.

CareMaps have a further advantage of placing the care in context. For example, before our system introduced CareMaps, the state department of health (DOH) would visit periodically and review the medical records. DOH reviewers usually found that patient weight was missing from a number of charts, and the hospital would receive deficiencies. Quality management staff attempted to educate the nurses on the importance of entering weight on the chart, and administrators even purchased new scales, but nothing improved. Weighing patients is important. Medication has to be calculated according to weight. In heart failure patients a weight gain can signal a serious problem; therefore a baseline weight is essential for effective treatment. When simply part of the normal routine, it is easy to neglect recording weight during the history and physical. Perhaps it doesn't seem critical to the patient's health and well-being. But when weight is part of a clinical context, as it is in the CareMap for heart failure, nurses respond and the weights get entered. Recording the weight stops being a mindless and meaningless chore and instead becomes integral to the treatment plan.

The CareMap provides a clinical background for why things are done the way they are done. It requires that the nurse record the medication so that the next caregiver knows what the patient received and with what outcome. In today's health care system many specialists and consultants are involved in a single patient's care, but no one has the time or patience to shuffle through a collection of everyone else's disorganized progress notes. A tool like a CareMap, which allows everyone to see the daily treatment quickly and simply, eliminates errors.

The CareMap also encourages accountability; everything is oriented to the patient. If something is missing or has been overlooked, a reminder is right there on the CareMap. These reminders are quite useful. No one can remember everything. A busy nurse handles about eight patients; a busy doctor may be treating fifty patients. CareMaps provide useful reminders to the physician and nursing staff.

CASE EXAMPLE:
DETOXIFICATION GUIDELINES

The following example illustrates the value of guideline development for improving patient safety and avoiding serious events. Aggregated data from our system's quality management sentinel event database alerted leadership that there had been several incidences of patient suicide and attempted suicides. These events occurred not solely in the behavioral health setting but, surprisingly, in the acute care setting as well. Perhaps because these medical and surgical patients arrived at the hospital for medical rather than for psychological problems, their underlying behavioral health issues remained undiagnosed.

To address the problem of inpatient suicide, a multidisciplinary task force—with members drawn from the medical staff and nursing staff and from the environmental services, pharmacy, quality management, risk management, social services, and ancillary departments in the system's community and tertiary hospitals—was formed to develop guidelines for assessing potential suicides. Over a period of several years, members of the task force interviewed staff, researched the relevant literature, and analyzed the medical record associated with each suicide incident.

The following case history is a composite of actual cases, and it illustrates some of the deficits in identifying and treating suicidal patients. Root cause analysis of cases such as this helped to target areas for improvement and the development of guidelines.

A fifty-four-year-old male was admitted to the ED with gastrointestinal bleeding. He was transferred from the ED to the medical intensive care unit (MICU), where he received transfusions and medication. A scan located the source of the bleeding, and after being stabilized he was discharged from the MICU and transferred to a medical patient care unit. Because the patient showed agitation and was wandering the halls, he was placed on one-to-one observation. Nonetheless, he entered the nursing station and demanded to use the phone and to smoke. Security was called to escort him back to his room. Once there, he became increasingly agitated, pulled out his IV lock, and was aggressive when the nurse attempted to take his vital signs and to give him medication. The patient was placed on wrist restraints which he quickly broke out of. He then shattered the window in his room with his roommate's IV pole, jumped out of the window, and died.

In order to examine the factors that contributed to this suicide, members of the task force created a time line, reflecting what happened when, and developed a cause and effect diagram to identify processes and issues that might have influenced this tragic outcome. These specific issues and processes were categorized into larger groupings: patient assessment, the environment, interventions, staff, and policies and procedures. From this information and through meetings of relevant staff and experts over a period of weeks, risk points were identified, illustrating where the care had broken down.

In this example the patient was not adequately assessed, and therefore the caregiving staff missed the signs and symptoms of alcohol withdrawal, a syndrome known to be associated with increased risk of suicide. Adequate assessment would have alerted the staff to the significance of the heightened agitation, and then appropriate medical management might have prevented this tragedy. In addition, the nursing and resident staff had not communicated the patient's escalating behavioral symptoms to the attending physician.

As a result of these findings, a multidisciplinary alcohol detoxification protocol development committee was convened to research and adopt an objective instrument to improve and standardize the identification of medical and surgical patients with alcohol problems and to enhance the medical management of patients undergoing alcohol withdrawal and at potential risk for suicide. The committee drew on the expertise of the medical, nursing, and psychiatric leadership throughout the system.

After nine months of research and planning, the alcohol detoxification protocol was designed, using evidence-based objective criteria, the CIWA-Ar (Clinical Institute Withdrawal Assessment-Alcohol, revised) scale, to evaluate the risk of alcohol withdrawal. The CIWA-Ar scale measures the extent of the anxiety, agitation, orientation, auditory, visual, and tactile disturbances typical of withdrawal symptoms. Interpretation of the scale objectifies withdrawal intensity, and on the basis of the evaluation medical management can be standardized. Clinical guidelines for patients assessed as at risk for alcohol withdrawal, with suggested physician order sets for treatment, were also developed from national guidelines and internal expertise. An alcohol detoxification treatment guideline in the form of a CareMap insert was incorporated into the primary CareMap of the acute care patient thought to be at risk.

The alcohol detoxification protocol, which included guidelines, education, and use of assessment tools, was reviewed and approved by the chairs of the departments of medicine and psychiatry, administration, and quality management, the associate chair for the Medical Intensive Care Unit, the multidisciplinary hospital performance improvement coordinating group, and chief residents. Although the approved policy was mandatory, its implementation required time and education. Recognizing that patients with this condition may be admitted to any service, the education and training program targeted nurses and physicians from surgery, maternity, and trauma as well as medicine.

Because these tools and protocols were new to the acute care medical and surgical units, educating the health care team about their use was necessary. Education was provided in a variety of medical and nursing forums to ensure appropriate patient assessment as well as initiation and maintenance of a medication regime upon the initial assessment or subsequent reassessment of a patient with actual or potential alcohol withdrawal. Classes for nursing staff included an overview of alcoholism, screening and assessment of patients at risk for withdrawal, use of the CIWA-Ar scale, and use of the CAGE questionnaire, a nonjudgmental tool to evaluate the patient's use of alcohol. Several system hospitals incorporated the topic into medical staff grand rounds.

A suicide, attempted or completed, is such a harrowing experience for the professional staff that staff members were committed to learning whatever they could to prevent such an incident from occurring. Once the initial unfamiliarity was overcome, the new protocol was embraced, and there were many requests for on-site education at specific hospital units. Through clinicians' greater awareness of the connection between alcohol withdrawal and the potential for suicide in the acute care setting and through increased communication between patient and caregiver, an improved therapeutic environment was created.

SUMMARY

To promote quality internally, the organization has to be committed to

- Developing quality databases to monitor the delivery of care.
- Adopting quality management methodologies to improve the delivery of care.

- Educating staff about quality management methods.
- Developing multidisciplinary teams to develop, promote, and implement clinical guidelines.
- Using CareMaps, or clinical pathways, to standardize care across different levels of treatment and across different health care facilities.
- Using CareMaps to improve documentation of treatment and outcomes.
- Using CareMaps to improve communication among caregivers.
- Reducing resource consumption and expenditure through CareMap methodology.
- Educating patients about their treatment through information, such as provided on a patient friendly CareMap.
- Documenting and analyzing variation from the outlined standard of care.

Things to Think About

You are in a leadership position in your hospital, and data reveal that the majority of physicians do not comply with evidence-based guidelines. Your job is to convince them to change. How would you do it?

- How would you analyze the problem?
- What data would you use to try and influence their behavior?
- What consequences (financial and clinical) would you bring to their attention?
- What would you do if the behavior did not change?

CHAPTER NINE

Using Data
for Performance
Improvement

A mong the many challenges that face health care administrative leadership is encouraging community physicians to abide by hospital regulations. Even those physicians who receive stipends or salaries to direct services often don't acknowledge the value of implementing regulatory requirements. For many of them, regulations are "just paper" and more of an annoyance than an important and legitimate way to monitor the process of care or to benefit the organization. However, because compliance is required by regulatory agencies—for example, hospitals must meet the expectations of the CMS (Centers for Medicare and Medicaid Services) core measures when providing assessment and treatment and comply with the IHI (Institute for Healthcare Improvement) initiative that focuses on reducing infection with preventive behavior such as hand washing—administrators need to find a way to convince physicians that all the hospital's rules matter. Modern medical care requires a kind of resocialization, a new mind-set, through which caregivers realize that measures are not designed to be an end in themselves but to be a means to improve the way medical care is implemented. When quality data are presented in such a way that physicians can see the benefit of using measures to evaluate and improve care, physicians become more willing to incorporate quality methodology into the way they practice.

The best way to mediate between meeting the requirements of the regulatory agencies and physicians' desire to manage patient care independently is to use data from specifically defined measures to prove that care can be evaluated, benchmarked for comparison, and improved. In this chapter I will present several performance improvement initiatives, examples based on initiatives conducted in our health care system. Each of the following examples illustrates how the use of data and measurements, combined with a deliberate performance improvement methodology, successfully improved patient safety, organizational performance, and financial expenditure. Through collaboration among clinical disciplines and administrative, financial, and quality departments, these performance improvement initiatives have standardized the delivery of care across different levels of care and across the continuum of care. These initiatives, published in quality journals and presented in quality forums, have become models of best practice across the country.

AGGREGATED DATA OFFER A DIFFERENT PERSPECTIVE

Performance improvement addresses classes of patients and wrestles with important questions that have to do with professional and clinical accountability and administrative ability to provide effective and efficient care. For example, do surgery patients have infections, and if so, what kind? Are some surgeries less infection prone than others, and if so, why? What are the consequences of the infections, to the patient and to the organization? Is there a class of patients, such as the elderly, who are more susceptible to infections, and if so, what improvements can be made? Without data, these questions can be answered only by guesswork and trial and error.

Measures help physicians focus on the risks their patients face, from the environment, from the treatment, and from disease complications. Measures also help administrative and health care leaders organize and plan for the most effective and efficient processes—those that have the best outcome on the highest volume of patients. For physicians, who are busy and pressured and trained to work alone, proactive, that is, preventive, maintenance for an entire class of patients may seem like an organizational responsibility rather than a clinical activity. But it isn't. Evidence shows that the majority of patients with pneumonia who receive an antibiotic in the first four hours of admittance to the hospital have better outcomes than those who don't. Then why not take the approach that all pneumonia patients should get a timely and appropriate antibiotic unless contraindicated for some clinical reason? Everyone wants good results.

Planning for improvement is necessary because a complex hospital environment may be difficult to monitor. Crowded conditions in the emergency department (ED) may create obstacles to identifying proper interventions for patients quickly. The triage process may be influenced by communication (or lack thereof) with the attending physicians. Radiological studies may turn over slowly. Staff may be limited, and competency issues may be involved in appropriate and timely assessment.

CASE EXAMPLE: USING QUALITY METHODS TO ENSURE CONSISTENCY OF CARE

This example of an emergency medical service (EMS) performance improvement initiative illustrates how integrating quality methods into every level of care, including the ambulance service, can lead to improved clinical and organizational performance. Also, as I hope will be apparent, because the members of the EMS came to understand measures, and knew what they were measuring and why, they gained a sense of the role they play in the entire spectrum of care. Through their participation in the quality management structure, they realized how aggregated information leads to improvements.

Imagine the following scenario. At 11:05 A.M., a fifty-two-year-old male calls 911 complaining of chest pain and shortness of breath. The advanced life support ambulance stationed at the local community hospital, which is affiliated with our health system, is dispatched. The paramedics assess, treat, and transport the patient back to the local community hospital, arriving at 11:35 A.M. The emergency department staff assess, treat, and stabilize the patient, but the attending physician determines that the patient needs a higher level of care, care available only at the health system's tertiary center. At 12:05 P.M. the cardiologist at the tertiary hospital's cardiac catheterization lab, having decided that the patient needs an emergent coronary angiogram and possible angioplasty, notifies the system's interfacility EMS that a "cardiac rescue" is required. The EMS dispatch center activates the rescue protocol, immediately assigning the closest health system mobile intensive care unit. Upon their prompt arrival at the community hospital, the critical care paramedics evaluate and prepare the patient for transport. At 12:50 P.M., while en route to the tertiary center, the paramedics monitor the patient and send a twelve-lead electrocardiogram (EKG) to the waiting cardiologist via radio. Upon arrival at the tertiary hospital's catheterization lab, the paramedics give a report to the staff and transfer the care of the patient over to the cardiology team. At 1:35 P.M. the patient receives a coronary angiogram and subsequent angioplasty with a stent.

Before the initiative to improve emergency services, this critical patient would not have received this timely, efficient, and lifesaving care.

Several years ago system leadership realized the necessity of supplying all hospitals in the system with a well-trained emergency medical service so that there would be a link among facilities and the continuum of care could be maintained during ambulance transport. The performance improvement initiative had several goals. By collecting reliable and accurate data on patient flow, administrators would better understand the needs assessment for different facilities, and with an effective and efficient EMS, operating costs for transportation could be greatly reduced. Crucially, patient safety would be improved if the level of care were consistent and appropriate during transport. Leadership incorporated quality management methods and performance improvement standards into the EMS initiative, making the service accountable for maintaining patient information data and for developing measures to monitor and improve patient care.

The first step of any improvement project is to ascertain current practice. Therefore data on current and projected ambulance transportation needs were collected from all hospitals within the system, analyzed, and submitted to the administration for review and action. Administrators considered cost, availability of service, quality of service, liability, and other factors before determining that expanding the existing EMS would be the most efficient and effective way to provide a high level of service. By expanding the service, the system would have a link that would reach out to the community, extending the care provided within the doors of its hospitals to patients throughout the region. This expanded service would also be able to collect data that would track patient flow throughout the system facilities.

Improving the existing system required resource expenditure. EMS staff were trained on collecting and tracking data and on using retrospective chart review to monitor types of calls. More vehicles and associated equipment were purchased, and more than forty additional EMS employees were hired. Leaders committed resources to establish a viable headquarters, and resources were also allocated to establish a state-of-the-art dispatch and communications center as well as to install global positioning technology in EMS vehicles to encourage the most efficient use of the EMS fleet.

As the expanding EMS became more integrated into the systemwide performance improvement program, it developed its own table of measures to track specific patient and unit information and identify best practices as patients moved within the system.

A committee—composed of Center for Emergency Medical Services (CEMS) administrators, supervisors, division specialists, staff members, the CEMS medical director, and a representative of the system's department of quality management—met to develop strategies and to monitor improvements. Appropriate measures of care and thresholds that defined good care were developed collaboratively by the EMS medical director, administrators, and operations leadership. The measures tracked data about access to needed care and services, as well as the movement of patients from one site to another.

Information was collected that identified the specific unit or floor the patient was coming from and the specific location the patient was being brought to (pediatric ICU, neonatal ICU, cardiac catheterization lab, nursing home, and so forth). These data were later used to evaluate services in the community hospitals; hospital administrators also used them for strategic planning purposes. Other measurements included monitoring the timeliness of transports and the patient diagnoses (such as trauma, chest pain/cardiology, or respiratory distress).

Here are some examples of quality indicators collected by the EMS:

- Volume, type, and severity assessments of illness or injury in the patients transported by ambulance
- Whether medical evaluation is provided in a timely and appropriate manner
- Assurance that the transporting crew delivers the appropriate level of care

- Reliability of the accuracy and completeness of documentation
- Cooperation and integration with system departments and with other hospitals and EMS agencies in the identification and correction of problems that interfere with appropriate prehospital patient care
- Prenotification of accurate patient diagnosis, which enhances the rapid initiation of appropriate treatment protocols at the receiving hospital

The data collection efforts influenced operational decisions and improved patient safety. For example, New York State mandates a thirty-minute response time for patients using neonatal intensive care unit transports. Tracking this time allowed the EMS service to identify areas where improvement was necessary. The response time for these highly vulnerable patients then decreased. Also, the tracking of patient diagnoses revealed that 72 percent of advanced life support ambulance calls were for cardiac patients, and 2 percent of patients were transported for obstetrical service. Owing to this information, new programs were developed to educate staff, and appropriate equipment was purchased.

EMS data gave community hospitals more detailed information about the types of patients they were not able to care for. This information, in turn, helped administrators and planners to make intelligent and informed service expansion decisions. The information revealed where resources needed to be deployed and what types of resources were needed at each of the different facilities. For example, assessments could be made about how many basic life support and how many advanced life support ambulances needed to be stationed at each facility. From data collected on diagnosis-specific volume, targeted education could be developed. After data identified a 50 percent increase in cardiac rescue volume over an eight-month period, cardiac specialists responded by training staff via case conferences on cardiac rescues. Quality measures such as mortality, time for pediatric intensive care unit transport, time for neonatal intensive care unit transport, and time spent at sending facility also depend on diagnosis-specific volume.

Clinical and operational improvements were implemented as a result of analysis of the data. For example, one system hospital became aware that it was transferring approximately forty cardiology patients per month to a tertiary center for cardiac catheterization procedures. Given these data, administrative leaders realized the value of applying for a certificate for a cardiac catheterization unit in their own facility. Today the hospital has its own diagnostic catheterization lab and has increased the services it can provide to the community while simultaneously decreasing the proportion of patients it needs to transfer to a tertiary facility. Without the EMS data collection effort, this aggregated information would have remained unknown.

At the system level the aggregated information helped with planning strategies and led to more efficient use of system and hospital resources. For example, the cardiac catheterization lab at one of the tertiary centers increased its physical plant threefold and its procedure volume fourfold based on the EMS's ability to transport patients from the community hospitals to the tertiary facility. The health system was also able to significantly expand its rehabilitation centers because the expanded EMS service was able to move patients between facilities more efficiently than before. The improvement reduced the hospital length of stay (LOS) for orthopedic patients by two days.

One example of how dramatically clinical care was influenced by collecting EMS measurements concerns the three thousand patients with a diagnosis of acute myocardial infarction that our health care system receives annually. The vice president of cardiac services for the system found that data showed the ability to transfer patients to the cardiac catheterization lab in a timely fashion by using the rescue protocol had reduced the mortality rate significantly. Hospitals that have emergency transportation supporting a cardiac catheterization unit have a mortality rate of 3 percent, whereas those without it have a mortality rate of 11 percent. That's a significant difference. The data collection and performance improvement efforts have also lowered resource consumption. The LOS for coronary bypass patients with catheterization has been reduced by one day.

The structure of the EMS is based on a military model, with uniforms, clear responsibilities, and an established and respected hierarchy. Unlike other hospital departments, the EMS is directly involved with local and national law enforcement agencies. The director understands the value of the quality management model for performance improvement and knows that data provide information for a superior organization.

Through increasing its size and participating in the performance improvement methodology, the EMS became able to supply efficient service to all system hospitals, provide a link among facilities, maintain the continuum of care during ambulance transport, collect data on patient flow, develop and share a meaningful information system based on transportation data collected, and incorporate quality and performance improvement standards into the EMS system. Since the implementation of this initiative, clinical, organizational, and financial improvements have been made.

CASE EXAMPLE:
INCREASING ACCESS TO CARE

Our health system is committed to providing outstanding care to everyone who lives in its service area, regardless of ability to pay. However, this worthy goal is not easily achieved. Many factors need to be addressed before a community avails itself of health services. Understanding the complexities involved and analyzing the services rendered can lead to improvements that, again, benefit the patients, the hospital, and the physicians.

The following example of a deliberate performance improvement effort focuses on ambulatory care patients. Ambulatory patients are different from hospital inpatients in that the caregivers and the organization have little control over their treatment and thus the outcomes of that treatment. This improvement effort illustrates how much good can be accomplished when clinicians work together to improve care, using data to understand the areas that require improvement and then monitoring that the improvement efforts are sustained.

The Family Practice Ambulatory Care Center, a clinic affiliated with one of the community hospitals in our health system, determined to offer the local residents improved access to care by developing strategies that would address the special needs of the community served. Family practice is the medical specialty that provides comprehensive primary medical care regardless of a patient's age or sex or the nature of his or her illness.

To provide equal opportunity care, significant cultural, linguistic, economic, and social barriers had to be recognized and overcome. The focus of the initiative was to develop processes that would bring reluctant patients into care, and once they were there, convince them that the health system was responsive enough to their needs to keep them returning for follow-up and preventive care.

The region that the community hospital serves encompasses people from such varied geographical regions as Central America, Italy, China, and Russia. In the past few years the proportion of patients who are Spanish-speaking increased to almost 80 percent. To respond to this linguistic change, the family practice increased its bilingual staff significantly.

However, language was only one of the barriers that had to be overcome before the community felt comfortable using the health system. Many of the patients in the hospital service area are undocumented residents, which raised challenges such as lack of money, transportation, and insurance; fear of being reported to immigration; transience; and the effect all these stressors impose on families and individuals. To confront these problems the hospital leadership empowered the front-line staff to analyze, identify, and implement improvements.

Although the practice had subjective and anecdotal notions of its strengths and weakness and of the special needs of its patients, objective data were necessary to determine where to target quality improvement efforts. A multidisciplinary team that included representatives from all levels of the practice collaborated on the initiative. However, collecting accurate and complete data on quality in this ambulatory care setting was especially difficult because the data sets available for the inpatient setting had never been implemented in this setting. Even ambulatory care financial data did not capture the kind of data that the inpatient data did. Therefore new processes of data collection needed to be developed.

To measure the quality of care provided in this setting, the health system's quality management department developed a table of measures (see Table 9.1) to begin to capture both administrative data, like volume and appointment compliance, and clinical data on preventive health care indicators, like immunization of two-year-olds, Pap smears, and mammograms. Clinical data were obtained through a review of randomly selected medical charts appropriate to a specific indicator. These data and similar reports from ambulatory practices in other health system hospitals are sent to system quality management and are benchmarked both internally within the system and externally with other databases and Healthy People 2010 goals. These data helped the family practice clinic identify gaps in its delivery of care and opportunities for improvement.

Facility	Indicators	Compliance—2004				
		Q1	Q2	Q3	Q4	Total
Hospital X	Total visits					
	Total appointments scheduled					
	Appointment compliance (%)					
	New patients					
	Revisits					
	No-show rate (%)					
	Immunization of 2-year-olds					
	Mammograms					
	Pap tests					

Table 9.1. Sample Ambulatory Services Table of Measures.

Healthy People 2010 is a national initiative of defined health objectives intended to improve the health status and quality of life of Americans over the first decade of the new century and to eliminate disparities of care among different segments of the population. The objectives were drawn from health initiatives of the past several decades, including the Surgeon General's report titled *Healthy People 2000: National Health Promotion and Disease Prevention Objectives,* which established national health objectives and served as the basis for the development of state and community plans to improve health. The goals of the Healthy People 2010 initiative were developed through consensus among scientists and medical experts throughout the country, with the participation of more than 350 national health, state health, mental health, substance abuse, and environmental agencies and over eleven thousand public comments gathered from an interactive Web site. Measures have been developed to monitor improvements over time.

Unlike the EMS initiative, the ambulatory setting used no special technology or systems to improve access to care, and therefore no special costs were incurred for implementing improvements. For example, data revealed that the rate of appointment compliance was low. Not keeping appointments is a quality as well as an organizational issue because missed appointments have an impact on follow-up care, preventive care, and the ability of the practice to provide continuity of care with a specific provider. Appointment compliance is also important so that valuable appointment time is not wasted.

To address this problem, receptionists began calling to remind patients of upcoming appointments or to follow up on missed appointments, which were then rescheduled. The idea was to help patients understand that the practice cares about them and wants to provide the health care they require. When a patient was seen for a test or condition that required another visit, the nurse would take the time to explain the reasons for the new visit and would make sure the appointment was scheduled before the patient left the clinic. Considerable effort was made to define and accommodate the patient's specific impediment (such as work schedule, transportation, or child-care issues) to keeping an appointment.

Financial problems were also keeping patients away. Because most of the patients were not covered by insurance, either because they were undocumented or because they were above the income level for Medicaid, the hospital developed a sliding fee scale so that patients could pay according to ability. When Child Health Plus, a program that insures the pediatric population from birth to eighteen years of age, became available through the state, the family practice clinic became providers under that program and allocated clinic space to the insurance representative to make it convenient for families to enroll in the program. Children under eighteen represented approximately 20 percent of the total visits for the practice, so enabling their insurance was critical.

To serve the needs of the prenatal patients, the practice became associated with the Prenatal Care Assistance Program (PCAP). PCAP provides coverage for women through pregnancy, delivery, and postnatal care and includes care for the newborn child. Most important, for this population, PCAP does not exclude undocumented residents. The family practice clinic also facilitated the on-site presence of staff from the Special Supplemental Nutrition Program for Women, Infants, and Children (WIC), to expedite the sign-up process for new mothers.

In an effort to improve communication between the hospital and the community, strong efforts at community outreach became an essential part of the family practice residency program. Outreach included providing education to schools, senior citizen centers, and other organizations, and participating in health fairs. The program provided adult health screenings on blood pressure, thyroid disease, oral cancer, and bone density. Stations were set up with educational materials for the entire family on topics such as diabetes; drug and tobacco control; colon, prostate, and breast cancers; nutrition; preconception health; prenatal care; and breast self-examination. Outreach also involved visiting local churches and community centers to let people know about the services available through the family practice.

The staff understood that the largely foreign population did not come in for preventive health care but only when something was wrong. The women's health program began to strongly emphasize prevention through encouraging routine Pap smears and mammograms. To make sure the patients understood proper follow-up, the nurses developed the Pap Educational Form (in Spanish and English), which was provided at the time of exam. This form included the name of the physician, the date of the follow-up appointment, and an explanation that the patient could expect to receive a letter, both registered and through the regular mail, if a follow-up appointment was required. The staff knew such an explanation was important; they were sensitive to the fears of their patients about getting official mail about their immigration status. Also, in order to ensure that all children were fully immunized by two years of age, the charts of children under two were reviewed for immunization status at every visit. This effort resulted in 100 percent compliance with immunization requirements for two-year-olds.

The success of the program is reflected in data that show the high percentage of revisits in the total appointments scheduled, and the increased percentage of patients keeping appointments. The entire pediatric population of the practice is insured, with coverage that includes medical care, dental care, eye care, hospitalization, and a prescription plan. Also, because these children are receiving ongoing care at the family practice, rather than episodic care in an emergency department (the more common mode for the uninsured), they are able to get appropriate preventive care, as is reflected by the high rate of fully immunized children.

Complex problems require multipronged solutions. With hospital leadership's commitment to meet the challenges of their changing community and to support the staff of the family practice group in analyzing, identifying, and implementing improvements, patients are now able to negotiate multiple barriers to access compassionate quality health care. The improvements attained through this initiative have been sustained and are monitored through quarterly reports to quality management. The table of measures, the process of data collection, and the quality management methodology and structure were key to the family practice's success. Sharing data led to the establishment of best practices, decreased professional isolation in the ambulatory settings, prioritized communication among different disciplines, and educational programs for residents.

CASE EXAMPLE: IMPROVING STERILIZATION ACROSS THE SYSTEM

Performance improvement programs are begun for various reasons, among them serious events that call into question existing practices. What is particularly interesting about the following example of an improvement effort is that the focus of the improvement was not clinicians or other members of the caregiving team but staff who worked largely unnoticed to support patient safety. I am using this example to illustrate how performance improvement efforts are useful at every level of the organization.

The relationship between sterilization and infection makes identifying problems in sterilization a critical patient safety issue. Two incidents that involved poor sterilization processes in the operating room provoked the health system to implement a performance improvement initiative to target existing sterile processing procedures and develop a more comprehensive and standardized approach to employee competency.

A system sterilization committee, including clinical and nonclinical personnel with expertise in decontamination, disinfection, and sterilization, was formed to ascertain current practices and recommend improvements. The committee included representatives from infection control, perioperative services, sterile processing/central sterile, dentistry, materials management, and quality management. System employees were also represented, as were local, statewide, and national professional organizations.

The objectives of the initiative were to provide a centralized approach to sterile processing, improve quality, use labor and nonlabor resources efficiently, and develop defined standards of practice. To facilitate standardization the committee recommended that a centralized, dedicated area be responsible for the supervision of sterilization activities and for the control and maintenance of all the equipment needed for patient care. Before the improvement effort, sterilization activities, such as decontamination, preparation and packaging, basin and tray assembly, quality control validation, and equipment distribution, were conducted in various departments throughout the hospital. There was no centralized oversight or administrative accountability.

The goals of the performance improvement effort were to

- Improve the efficiency and processes involved in sterilization.
- Establish quality practices that meet sterilization standards and regulatory agency requirements.
- Develop a competent workforce through ongoing education.
- Redesign work processes to increase efficiency and optimize resource utilization.
- Provide technology and an environment conducive to optimal outcomes.
- Enhance patient satisfaction.

The scope of service included twenty-four-hour, seven-day coverage. An equipment assessment was conducted to ensure that state-of-the-art equipment was being used. An inventory of instrument trays was undertaken to understand and improve equipment throughout. In an effort to standardize job responsibilities and job competencies, a new staffing model was developed and a new staffing organization plan was created.

A subcommittee of certified central service managers and infection control and quality management staff reviewed all existing policies and procedures and developed new ones as deemed necessary. During the review of these documents, the subcommittee continued to consider the offerings of state-of-the-art vendors, including surgical instrument tracking systems and various products for decontamination, high-level disinfection, and sterilization. A vendor presentation at the system level provided current data from outside the system and fostered dialogue among the system central services managers about the propagation of best practice.

Another subcommittee addressed establishing a minimum credentialing standard. An inventory of staff education and competency led to the conclusion that many employees had been assigned to their positions in central processing with mostly on-the-job training and little formal education about sterilization. Only a small percentage of employees were certified through nationally accepted programs. Because the level of education, including the ability to read and write English, was inconsistent, a basic education program for sterile processing staff was created. This program was developed by a registered nurse with a background in education, assisted by certified central service managers, to support the competency of all employees involved with sterile processing. The program encompasses six standardized educational modules: infection control, decontamination and disinfection, sterile packing and storage, instrumentation, sterilization, and quality monitoring in the sterilization process. It serves as a minimum educational requirement for all central services and sterile processing staff involved with sterilization activities.

The employee is expected to achieve a passing score of 85 percent in each module. A knowledge and skills checklist is used to document the employee's completion of each module's learning objectives. All employees involved with sterilization and validation activities are expected to successfully complete the basic education program for sterile processing staff.

A technical training program was also implemented. Education in this program is provided by an outside source and sponsored by the hospital. Staff members, those responsible for the actual process of sterilization, the monitoring and documenting of the process, and adherence to regulatory agency standards, will be able to sit for the international certification exam.

The basic education program was approved by the health system's board of trustees and the medical boards; supervision is the responsibility of the managers of central services at the hospitals. Approximately 73 percent of the central service and sterile processing staff across the system are now registered or certified by a nationally recognized organization, such as the International Association of Health Care Central Service Materials Management and the National Institute for the Certification of Healthcare Sterile Processing and Distribution Personnel. Prior to the implementation of this program, only three staff members in the health system were certified.

Formalizing the sterilization process increased professionalism and raised a sense of worth and pride among the workforce. As appropriate, individuals have been "grandfathered" into their positions, based on a basic knowledge assessment and demonstrated competency.

COLLABORATION WORKS

Improvements such as the ones I have described in these three examples are dependent on many levels of the organization working collaboratively together and relying on objective data to identify problems and monitor solutions to those problems. To provide the best care and improve patient outcomes, cooperation among administrators, quality management staff, and clinical staff is most successful. Each group learns from the other. Utilization measures, generally thought to be administrative tools, inform the physician about the efficiency of the care provided. Quality measures target gaps in the delivery of care, measuring the difference between the evidence and the practice.

Due to the pressure imposed by the CMS for compliance with quality measures, physicians are beginning to take responsibility for more than their specialty. It used to be that a busy cardiac surgeon would perform the surgery, then leave. His or her responsibility began and ended in the operating room, leaving the supervision of the pre-op and post-op care to others. Data reveal that pre- and post-op care have an impact on adverse events and complications, whereas consistency of supervision helps to eliminate problems. For example, when blood thinners are not stopped before the surgery, bleeds and other serious complications occur. These are problems that can be easily solved with appropriate supervision of the entire care process, not just a single piece of it. By analyzing measures, the cardiac surgeons realized that the entire continuum of care had an impact on whether surgical outcomes were successful or unsuccessful. The measures that were collected addressed the issues related to the causes of poor outcomes, and they revealed that the pre- and post-op care made the difference between life and death.

Hospitals support organizational measures because they need to monitor their provision of care and services. If they need to change processes to be more efficient, then they do. But unless there is an objective standard against which to benchmark, it is difficult to know when, or what, to improve. When physicians, rather than functioning in isolated groups or sometimes even antagonistic ones, participate with administrators in quality management activities to develop and encourage the use of measures, clinical and organizational processes improve.

Because measures are objective and used for improvements, agencies that develop them are responsive to clinical input. For example, CMS changed a measure associated with coronary artery bypass graft (CABG) surgery when a medical society took issue with it because it focused on stopping prophylactic antibiotics for CABG procedures within forty-eight hours postsurgery. When the medical society showed data, that is, evidence, that seventy-two hours of treatment and a different antibiotic were superior to the treatment associated with the measure, the measure was changed. Working together benefits everyone.

When a doctor has a solo practice, as many do, he or she is entirely in charge of the patient's destiny. Moreover physicians have the most intimate access to their patients. It is easy to see why so many physicians feel the intense responsibility to take charge and why they might resist being told what to do by anyone. Nonetheless, they need to be persuaded that incorporating measures, and aggregated data, into the way they practice can serve them and their patients well. Therefore, when the data show that their patients have an inappropriately and unnecessarily long LOS or a higher infection rate than the national benchmark, they have open minds and examine their process of care and see where and how to improve. Slowly, the data and the improved results from complying with the measures are making a difference and influencing care.

SUMMARY

Performance improvement data improve clinical, organizational, and financial processes through

- Exposing physicians to objective measures that assess the delivery of care.
- Providing data that lead to improved processes.
- Monitoring and standardizing care across the continuum.
- Exposing caregivers and administrators to the results of aggregated data.
- Identifying risk points and gaps in care for defined populations.

- Targeting proactive strategies to benefit particular patient populations.
- Bringing various disciplines together to collaborate on quality management processes.
- Accurately assessing current practices and identifying inefficient processes.
- Providing information about the most effective expenditure of resources.
- Enabling caregivers and health care leadership to track and trend the results of improvement efforts.
- Encouraging multidisciplinary communication.
- Influencing strategic planning decisions.
- Informing leadership about education deficits.
- Revealing efficiencies of resource allocation.
- Objectively assessing patient and community needs.

Things to Think About

You want to improve the care delivered in the high-risk environments in your hospital, such as the operating room, intensive care unit, emergency department, and chemotherapy unit.

- What processes would be the focus of your improvement efforts (for example, turnaround time in the OR)?
- How would you define your goals?
- What quality management methodology would you use to make these improvements?
- What questions would you ask? Of whom?
- Which departments or services would be involved?
- What variables would you monitor?
- What measures would you define?
- How would you check for improvements?
- How would you communicate the results of the improvement efforts?
- How would you evaluate the improvement efforts? For patients? For the organization?

—⌁— Conclusion

As I have repeatedly pointed out throughout the preceding chapters, the movement toward evaluating health care services through measurements is not only mandated by regulatory and governmental agencies and private, corporate, and community groups but should be embraced by clinicians and hospital leadership in order to promote the most effective and efficient processes of care. Measures help to ground clinical, operational, and financial decisions in objective facts, and aggregated data and publicly reported quality indicators should be considered meaningful yardsticks for defining good care.

Often physicians feel independent of the policies and procedures that the hospitals are required to follow. They want to do their job and not be interfered with. Some, in response to mandates to document the care they deliver, want to use technology, such as the computerized medical record, or want to hire people to do the documentation, physician assistants or nurse practitioners, so that they, the physicians, can be freed up to do the real work of healing. This attitude needs to change if health care is going to improve. Physicians need to participate in the process of improvement, not solely for their individual patients but for all patients, and this participation requires physicians to be convinced about the value of measuring care and documenting the process of care.

Administrative leadership tries all kinds of tricks to enlist physician support, mostly unsuccessfully. For example, many institutions develop checklists that require a simple yes or no checkmark. Even so, physicians and nurses don't perceive that these lists have any value in improving care. The challenge is to find a way to transform this mindset so that measures can be used proactively to shape changed practices. What I am suggesting is that buying fancy computers and software or developing simple checklists will not be enough to motivate professionals to use measures to understand and improve care— even when measures are required—only an internal change of culture will make a difference. My experience, over eighteen years in quality management, with 7,000 physicians in fourteen hospitals, outpatient clinics, and nursing homes, is that only a handful of these physicians are involved in primary quality management activities, such as conducting reviews, using data to analyze care, and participating in task forces to set standards.

There is a kind of Catch-22 involved: in order to show the need to improve care, it is necessary that physicians participate in data collection and documentation; yet physicians don't always see the value in this. They don't realize that the medical record has to be considered a coherent and legal database reflecting the patient's experience. Therefore they don't participate in data collection and documentation.

For measures to be used for improvement, they have to be taken seriously and not superficially. Even though the lessons of success are all around us, most U.S. industry, including the health care industry, doesn't stop to analyze small problems. Big industries hope they can get away without a major recall or a space flight disaster. But it makes more sense to ensure efficiency before a total recall or stoppage or public relations disaster occurs. In order to produce the best product possible—whatever it is—objective, valid, and reliable information is required, including comparative and competitive information. For health care that means statistics, data, measures, and benchmarks.

Physicians are not trained to think as industry leaders or to work collectively to benefit the organization they work in. Interestingly, many physicians see the value of working in groups to make the business end of their practice more efficient and cost effective. They share space and resources such as equipment and staff. Measures are accepted and used for certain aspects of business, but not for all. Physicians count how many patients they have, and how many patients miss appointments, for example, because it is important for their business that they know this information. In the same way, it is important to provide the most appropriate treatment for disease and to acknowledge aggregated wisdom, such as evidence-based measures, to improve care for a patient population.

Unfortunately, physicians also expect to work in isolation and are not always effective communicators. Traditionally they give orders and expect others to interpret and follow their instructions. Data show that such a style is not always the most effective way to work because the lack of communication among professional staff can result in problems. Particularly in today's health care organizations, with so many caregivers, specialists, consultants, and ancillary professionals interacting with an individual patient, it is often unclear who is managing the details and ensuring that instructions are carried out in a timely and efficient manner.

Communication must be not only productive but also measurable, so that instructions can be delivered to other care providers who interact with the patient. Everyone involved requires accurate statistics so that interventions don't contradict or adversely interact with other interventions. For example, a miscalculation or incorrect documentation of medication can lead to a drug reaction.

Part of the challenge involved in changing traditional modes of behavior is wrestling with the dichotomy between individual autonomy and collective cooperation. Measures reflect aggregated data and reveal commonalities about best practices. Physicians deal with individuals, and although they may agree in principle that evidence-based medicine is useful, they often perceive their particular patient as not typical. However, they do not need to rely on perception but to understand the statistical distance of their patients from the norm.

There is also a psychological factor to be addressed. Traditionally, physicians are in charge. They tell others what to do. Now, governmental agencies are telling them. This doesn't always go down easily. A habit of mind, or mind-set, resists change. Because measures are being introduced from areas external to the physician—the government, insurance companies, private purchasers of health care, or quality management departments—physicians think they are being controlled by outside sources and that the recommendations can be ignored.

When adverse events or incidents are analyzed, it is often the case that physicians did not make use of the appropriate, and readily available, algorithm of care or that they didn't communicate their thinking effectively to others involved with the patient and important information was lost. Mistakes, and sometimes very costly ones, occur for reasons unrelated to physician clinical competence. For example, a physician with a high volume of patients may not check, as required, the patient identification because he or she is rushed, or worse, arrogant. Mistakes happen, and the wrong patient gets the wrong procedure, blood, or medication. Avoidable errors should not occur. Many good doctors realize the likelihood of making a mistake if they are not very careful, and they are able to learn from the experience of others, use evidence-based guidelines appropriately, and insist on appropriate documentation in the medical chart so that everyone involved in the patient's care has the information needed. Measures that are valid and reliable, developed from severity- or risk-adjusted formulas to control for variation, have enormous explanatory and analytical force. What will improve hospital care and its efficiency and productivity is having more physicians join the ranks of those who are willing to use evidence-based guidelines to learn. Physicians, after all, hold the key to the mode of production (to use an industrial analogy) of a hospital. They bring in the patients, and they mold the product delivered to the patients. They control the application of labor and determine which resources are necessary to the provision of care.

To meet patient expectations, it is necessary to know what the national benchmarks are for achieving a high standard of care. Patients, no longer subservient to the all-knowing physician, expect to be treated correctly. They expect their care to conform to national norms. As scientists, physicians also rely on objective information, numbers, rates, and measures, to understand their individual patients. They should be able to accept collective measures as revealing of important aspects of care as well. Once a standard is accepted as the norm, deviations from the standard require analysis. It is a different way of thinking about providing care, but there are advantages.

Perhaps if administrative leaders stressed the bridge between, rather than the separation of, operational and clinical factors, physicians would follow their lead. As it presently stands, many administrators as well as many physicians view regulatory requirements as obstacles to doing their job. But these regulations, although crafted by sources external to the hospital, provide caregivers with high standards of care that should be embraced rather than reviled. Regulations are not "just paper," keeping the busy caregiver from providing bedside care. Regulations and documentation ensure that proper care is given and that communication is effective. Health care is a business, and using a business model to help change the mind-set of administrators and clinicians may be a good idea. Thinking about health care in terms of business accountability may be useful, because such an idea sees that measurements lead to profit for the patients in terms of recovery and long-term survival and for the organization in terms of economic margins, with a focus on productivity and efficiency.

The cultural gulf that now exists between the community and the hospital has to be bridged for health care to inspire confidence and for health care organizations to survive financially. The media often function as the community's representatives and have to be dealt with. Patients threaten hospitals with media exposure, which hospitals try to avoid. All this adversarial posturing does not build bridges. Hospitals need patients, physicians need patients, and it is important to try to build up trust. Although often resented, in fact the media help to hold hospitals accountable, and the community focuses national attention on safety. Both the media and community advocacy groups force change. Medical professionals have to shift from a traditional authoritarian posture to a more collaborative one. Quality objectives, methods, and data will help to transform the culture. Everyone shares the same agenda—safe care. And measures are seen as objective and unbiased toward any group. Objective methods reassure the community that there is oversight. Quality management programs should be seen as agents of change.

The next frontier for quality management is public education, including showing people how measures set by the Centers for Medicare and Medicaid Services (CMS) can be used to promote safety. The use of data and databases to evaluate hospitals and physicians can connect process measures with outcome measures. If, for example, a ninety-year-old patient with pneumonia is not given an antibiotic and that patient dies, sooner or later connections will be made. Communities are aware of the importance of preventive medicine, especially when the possibility of death is quantified.

Politically and socially, it seems as if the medical profession is reluctant to let the public into the secrets of its trade. This is the mindset that needs to be changed; it is more about protecting the caregiver than the patient. In my opinion, quality management should help to drive this change, teaching professionals and community groups alike to use and rely on data and measurements to analyze and evaluate care. Quality management can also educate caregivers about the importance of documentation, that it improves care and is not simply meaningless paperwork. Documentation becomes the database for evaluating what has occurred during a hospitalization. For many years there was no oversight of health care practices. When administrators stop thinking about quality management as an arm of the regulatory agencies and instead consider it a vital link between professional staff and patients, change will occur.

Traditionally, medical schools have trained physicians to consider the patient as an individual, not to look at aggregated data to understand a patient population and not to consider the organizational issues associated with an episode of hospitalization. Medical students are not taught to benefit from best practice guidelines or benchmarks or developing patient profiles for particular diagnoses. Therefore they are understandably unfamiliar with and somewhat resistant to using measures to understand their patients and their delivery of care.

But times are changing. Although quality management courses are being introduced for medical residents and also into the curricula of programs in health care administration, nursing, and public health, they are still not part of the medical school curriculum. Quality management methods and measures and regulatory requirements are most often considered operational or business issues rather than clinical issues. Such distinctions are antiquated and harmful in today's health care environment.

In China, where I was called upon to play a part in setting up that nation's health care system through teaching quality management to physicians and health care executives, officials are eager to do it the right way. Compared to Western habits, the prevalent mind-set in China is much less focused on individual performance and success and much more comfortable with the notion that doing good work collectively makes an organization run efficiently. The physicians understand that the business value of cooperation, as well as the organizational effectiveness of working together to achieve a high standard of care, is not removed from clinical performance.

The reasons to educate our own new physicians in quality management are numerous. Among them are to bridge the gap between what medical schools teach and the reality of health care practice, and to understand the regulatory framework in which physicians work, including meeting the expectations of evidence-based medicine. Physicians need education about the public reporting of data; they need to know that their educated patient, or consumer, may well research their compliance rate with physician-specific, publicly reported quality indicators.

New physicians are also not taught about the many regulatory and other forces to which they will be held accountable, such as complying with quality indicators from the Institute of Medicine (IOM), Joint Commission on Accreditation of Healthcare Organizations (JCAHO), and local departments of health (DOH) and from the CMS, HMOs, community advocacy groups, drug companies, and their own malpractice insurers. These groups are just the external forces they have to reckon with. Internally, the hospital that they affiliate with will require compliance as well. Medical schools are not doing their students a service when they leave those students to figure this out on the spot.

There is also a great deal of pressure from the media and other groups to standardize care, based on evidence-based indicators. Many beginning physicians don't even know about the research or the regulations or about such compelling organizational drivers of quality as pay-for-performance initiatives or financial incentives for hospitals. But when newspapers such as the *New York Times* publish data about how well regional hospitals are delivering appropriate care (as defined by CMS quality indicators) and these physicians are associated with one of the poorly performing hospitals, it is not going to please their patients.

In the health care system in which I work, residents, with the support of system leadership, receive education about quality management and the expectations of regulatory agencies through many forums. Quality management is part of resident orientation as are such special topics as the data published by the Agency for Healthcare Research and Quality (AHRQ) and JCAHO, the CMS indicators, and tracer methodology. Residents are also expected to participate in performance improvement initiatives. The health system has established a clinical rotation in quality management, at the request of the residents themselves, who realize how important it is to them to understand how to work within a quality framework. They receive hands-on experience with issues related to clinical performance measurement, patient safety, and internalizing quality methods into practice.

Today's quality management departments do more than conduct compliance and incident analysis and interface with regulatory bodies. They encourage and monitor the use of evidence-based medicine to establish uniform standards of care. Quality management collects data that reflect aggregated numbers; that define the scope of care of different patient populations and hospitals; that can compare treatment, interventions, and outcomes for various populations; that help to establish benchmarks for outcomes; and that monitor improvement efforts.

Health care organizations have no choice but to collect and analyze quality measures, because developing quality indicators for monitoring and improving health care processes is required by JCAHO, state DOHs, and the CMS, and these measures are used by the IOM and HMOs to analyze care. Therefore those involved with health care delivery and services must understand how to work within this framework and use quality data, not solely to meet regulatory requirements but also to reach a high level of organizational performance and financial success. This is no longer the wave of the future but the wave washing ashore right now.

In addition to quality management principles and methods, residents in our health care system learn about using data to evaluate processes, how control charts and outcomes analysis can help them understand their delivery of care, the importance of reporting errors and near misses, how to do incident analysis, and how to understand benchmarks and best practices—all with the goal of improving patient safety.

Rather than rely solely on physicians to monitor clinical services, an alternative, more effective leadership style is to attempt to understand the complexity of care and to evaluate it through collecting information, analyzing data, communicating with staff, and requiring appropriate personnel to be responsible for the safe, effective, and efficient delivery of care. This approach may be more arduous and effortful in the short run, but it will lead to greater clinical and operational successes in time. Unless leadership asks clinicians about their processes, their successes, and their failures, there will be no way to even understand, no less improve, the delivery of care. With information about volume, growth, areas of growth, changed practices, the organization's response to community needs, efficacy of equipment, services, staff, and so forth, leaders can equip themselves to make informed and effective decisions.

ᴕ Bibliography

Agency for Health Care Policy and Research (AHCPR). *Clinical Practice Guidelines No. 3.* Rockville, Md.: U.S. Department of Health and Human Services, 1994.

Aguayo, R. *Dr. Deming: The American Who Taught the Japanese About Quality.* New York: Simon & Schuster, 1990.

Annandale, E., Elston, M. A., and Prior, L. *Medical Work, Medical Knowledge and Health Care.* Malden, Mass.: Blackwell, 2004.

Berwick, D. M. "Continuous Improvement as an Ideal in Health Care." In N. O. Graham (ed.), *Quality in Health Care: Theory, Application, and Evolution.* Gaithersburg, Md.: Aspen, 1995.

Champy, J. *X-Engineering for the Corporation: Reinventing Your Business in the Digital Age.* New York: Warner Books, 2002.

Chowdhury, S. *The Power of Six Sigma.* Chicago: Dearborn, 2001.

Cockerham, W. C. *Medical Sociology.* Upper Saddle River, N.J.: Prentice Hall, 1989.

Codman, E. A. *A Study in Hospital Efficiency as Demonstrated by the Case Report of the First Five Years of a Private Hospital.* Oakbrook Terrace, Ill.: Joint Commission on Accreditation of Healthcare Organizations, 1996.

Colen, B. D. *O.R.: The True Story of 24 Hours in a Hospital Operating Room.* New York: Dutton, 1993.

Dlugacz, Y. D. Review of "Methods of Family Research: Biographies of Research Projects, Vol. II." *Readings: Journal of Reviews and Commentary in Mental Health,* May 1990.

Dlugacz, Y. D. "Handling a Surprise JCAHO Inspection." *Modern Healthcare,* Nov. 14, 2005, S10–S11.

Dlugacz, Y. D. "Keep It Clean!" *Health Care Link,* Aug. 23, 2005.

Dlugacz, Y. D., Restifo, A., and Greenwood, A. *The Quality Handbook for Health Care Organizations: A Manager's Guide to Tools and Programs.* San Francisco: Jossey-Bass, 2004.

Dlugacz, Y. D., Restifo, A., and Nelson, K. "Implementing Evidence-Based Guidelines and Reporting Results Through a Quality Metric." *Patient Safety and Quality Healthcare,* 2005, *2*(2), 40–42.

Dlugacz, Y. D., Rosati, R. J., and Tortolani, A. J. "Communicating Quality Assurance Data to Trustees." *Quality Times* (Hospital Association of New York State), Mar. 1991.

Dlugacz, Y. D., and Stier, L. "More Quality Bang for Your Healthcare Buck." *Journal of Nursing Care Quality,* 2005, *20,* 174–181.

Dlugacz, Y. D., Stier, L., and Greenwood, A. "Changing the System: A Quality Management Approach to Pressure Injuries." *Journal for Healthcare Quality,* 2001, *23*(5), 15–20.

Dlugacz, Y. D., and others. "Expanding a Performance Improvement Initiative in Critical Care." *Joint Commission Journal on Quality Improvement,* 2002, *28,* 419–434.

Dlugacz, Y. D., and others. "Safety Strategies to Prevent Suicide in Multiple Health Care Environments." *Joint Commission Journal on Quality and Safety,* 2003, *29,* 267–277.

Donabedian, A. "The Role of Outcomes in Quality Assessment and Assurance." In N. O. Graham (ed.), *Quality in Health Care: Theory, Application, and Evolution.* Gaithersburg, Md.: Aspen, 1995.

Gawande, A. *Complications: A Surgeon's Notes on an Imperfect Science.* New York: Metropolitan Books, 2002.

George, M. L. *Lean Six Sigma for Service.* New York: McGraw-Hill, 2003.

Halm, E. A., and others. "Limited Impact of a Multicenter Intervention to Improve the Quality and Efficiency of Pneumonia Care." *Chest,* 2004, *126,* 100–107.

Hussain, E., and Kao, E. "Medication Safety and Transfusion Errors in the ICU and Beyond." *Critical Care Clinics,* 2005, *21*(1), 91–110.

Joint Commission on Accreditation of Healthcare Organizations. *Framework for Improving Performance: From Principles to Practice.* Joint Commission Resources. Oakbrook Terrace, Ill.: Joint Commission on Accreditation of Healthcare Organizations, 1994.

Joint Commission on Accreditation of Healthcare Organizations. *Florence Nightingale: Measuring Hospital Outcomes.* Joint Commission Resources. Oakbrook Terrace, Ill.: Joint Commission on Accreditation of Healthcare Organizations, 1999.

Joint Commission on Accreditation of Healthcare Organizations. *Failure Mode and Effects Analysis in Health Care: Proactive Risk Reduction.* Joint Commission Resources. Oakbrook Terrace, Ill.: Joint Commission on Accreditation of Healthcare Organizations, 2002.

Joint Commission on Accreditation of Healthcare Organizations. *From Practice to Paper: Documentation for Hospitals.* Joint Commission Resources. Oakbrook Terrace, Ill.: Joint Commission on Accreditation of Healthcare Organizations, 2002.

Joint Commission on Accreditation of Healthcare Organizations. *Hospital Accreditation Standards.* Joint Commission Resources. Joint Commission on Accreditation of Healthcare Organizations, 2002.

Juran, J. M. *Juran on Quality by Design: The New Steps for Planning Quality into Goods and Services.* New York: Free Press, 1992.

Kohn, L. T., Corrigan, J. M., and Donaldson, M. S. (eds.). *To Err Is Human: Building a Safer Health System.* Washington, D.C.: National Academies Press, 1999.

Lustbader, D., Cooper, D., Reiser, P., Dlugacz, Y. D., and Fein, A. "Methodology for Improved ICU Resource Utilization and Quality of Care." *Chest,* 1998, *114,* 254S.

Lustbader, D., Dlugacz, Y. D., Weissman, G., Stier, L., and Fein, A. "Regional Benchmarking for Critical Care: Methodology for Quality Improvement." *Chest,* 1998, *114,* 342S.

Lustbader, D., Sparrow, P., Silver, A., Dlugacz, Y. D., and Fein, A. "Ventilator Care in a Large Hospital Network." *Chest,* 1998, *114,* 343.

McKinlay, J. B., Lin, T., Freund, K., and Moskowitz, M. "The Unexpected Influence of Physician Attributes on Clinical Decisions: Results of an Experiment." *Journal of Health and Social Behavior,* 2002, *43*(1), 92–106.

Milstein, A., and others. "Improving the Safety of Health Care: The Leapfrog Initiative. The Leapfrog Group." *Effective Clinical Practice,* 2000, *5,* 313–316.

The New England Journal of Medicine. *Quality of Care: Selections from the New England Journal of Medicine.* Waltham: Massachusetts Medical Society, 1997.

Parsons, T. *The Social System.* New York: Free Press, 1951.

Robertson, S., Lesser, M. L., Kohn, N., Cooper, D. J., and Dlugacz, Y. D. "Statistical and Methodological Issues in the Evaluation of Case Management Studies." *Journal of Health Care Quality,* 1996, *18*(6), 25–31.

Rosati, R., and Dlugacz, Y. D. *The Use of Data Analysis and Feedback to Manage the Length of Stay of Medically Treated Neurology Patients.* Philadelphia: Society for Medical Decision Making, 1991.

Siegel, C., Alexander, M. J., Dlugacz, Y. D., and Fischer, S. "Evaluation of a Computerized Drug Review System: Impact, Attitudes and Interactions." *Computers and Biomedical Research,* Oct. 1984, 419–434.

Spath, P. L. "Reducing Errors Through Work System Improvements." In P. L. Spath (ed.), *Error Reduction in Health Care: A Systems Approach to Improving Patient Safety.* San Francisco: Jossey-Bass, 2000.

Stier, L., and others. "Reinforcing Organization-Wide Pressure Ulcer Reduction on High-Risk Geriatric Inpatient Units." *Outcomes Management,* 2004, *8*(1).

Studer, Q. *Hardwiring Excellence: Purpose, Worthwhile Work, and Making a Difference.* Gulf Breeze, Fla.: Fire Starter, 2003.

Timmermans, S., and Angell, A. "Evidence-Based Medicine, Clinical Uncertainty, and Learning to Doctor." *Journal of Health and Social Behavior,* 2001, *42,* 342–359.

Weinstock, M. S., and Dlugacz, Y. D. "Integration of Emergency Department Care with the Hospital Process." In *Quality Assurance in Emergency Medicine.* (2nd ed.) Irving, Tex.: American College of Emergency Physicians.

White, K. *An Introduction to the Sociology of Health and Illness.* Thousand Oaks, Calif.: Sage, 2002.

Williams, S. C., Schmaltz, S. P., Morton, D. J., Koss, R. G., and Loeb, J. M. "Quality of Care in U.S. Hospitals as Reflected by Standardized Measures, 2002–2004." *New England Journal of Medicine,* 2005, *353,* 255–264.

Zussman, R. *Intensive Care: Medical Ethics and the Medical Profession.* Chicago: University of Chicago Press, 1992.

~~~ Index